RESILIENCE
—— IN THE FACE OF ——
MULTIPLE
SCLEROSIS

*"IT WILL MAKE A BIG DIFFERENCE AND BRING HOPE
TO MANY PEOPLE'S LIVES"*-MABEL KATZ

BRANDON BEABER, M.D.

Foreword by Sky-Ellen Beaber Ph.D.

Contributions by Rex Beaber J.D. Ph.D., Mark Katz Ph.D., Melissa Fledderjohann Ph.D., Jon Forsyth Ph.D., Mabel Katz

Edited by The Artful Editor, Rex Beaber J.D. Ph.D., Alice Handel, Dr. Alan Epstein, J.R. Alcoyne J.D., Calli, Shalom Rabizadeh, [fiverr.com accounts] gingermaneditor, thornecomm5r, kitd56

Proofread by Donna Rich

Cover Design by 100Covers.com
Interior Design by FormattedBooks.com

ISBN-13: 978-1-7332426-2-2
ISBN-10: 1-7332426-2-7

PRAISE FOR
RESILIENCE IN THE FACE OF MULTIPLE SCLEROSIS

"A unique exploration of this very important psychologic construct in persons with MS. The detailed and engrossing individual patient stories will resonate with readers, and there are clear explanations of practical strategies that can be used to develop and enhance resilience for anyone with a chronic illness.

—Barbara S. Giesser M.D., Author of *Multiple Sclerosis for Dummies*

Dr. Beaber shares the inspiring stories of five people who challenged his beliefs about what it means to live well with MS—an unpredictable and often disabling disease. As a young doctor, he takes us on his journey to see beyond the fear and physical disability MS can cause, to discover the power of resilience these remarkable individuals display. He introduces us to an in-depth, yet accessible overview of the often-confusing and seemingly conflicting theories of resilience. Throughout the book, he skillfully interweaves pragmatic ways all of us can improve our resilience. His compassionate voice shines through and will encourage you!

—Annette Langer-Gould M.D. Ph.D., Multiple sclerosis specialist and regional lead for Clinical and Translational Neuroscience for the Southern California Permanente Medical Group

"An amazing piece for patients to learn about things they have control over...a wakeup call to the medical community, that they are being cavalier about the process of accepting diagnoses. I love the whole shifting perspective, mindfulness, etc....it is well written with a unique insight...a great read."

—Marie Heron, Host of the Living with MS Truth be Told podcast, Qigong for MS instructor, speaker, and patient advocate

"If you are impacted by MS, then you need to read this book right now! I've learned a lot from reading it, lessons I look forward to sharing with my own clinic patients."

—Aaron Boster M.D., Systems medical chief of neuroimmunology & director MS center, OhioHealth.

"Beaber explores the personal stories of his patients dealing with MS, as well as other hardships. Dr. Beaber's expert synthesis of personal, medical, and psychological elements is powerful and inspiring. This academic work reminds us that we all have strength and courage within us to face life's challenges.

—Gail C Brady, M.D., Psychiatrist

"This manuscript is an amazing opportunity for education and growth on multiple fronts. It does a great job combining psychological frameworks for treating MS in a novel way. Resiliency is a powerful tool and is displayed beautifully."

—Melissa Fledderjohann Ph.D., Clinical psychologist and director of pain management at San Mateo Medical Center

"Open-minded in terms of what can help people, be it traditional religion or philosophy or Buddhist concepts and ideas."

—J.R. Alcyone, Author of *Five Fathoms Beneath*

"The author presents a very humanistic appreciation for his patients, tries to not define them by their MS, and yet also describes how they have integrated (and to what degree) their MS into their identity and self-concept. Emerging research has shown that resilience can be taught and enhanced through training and therapy. Therefore, resilience may be conceptualized as a skill that can be drawn upon and refined, even if individuals are born with more or less resilience at the outset. Presenting this perspective early on promotes hope and motivation of the reader to pursue activities to enhance their own resilience."

—Anonymous Academic Reviewer

"As a neurologist, treating patients with MS, I have encountered countless situations in which patients, after receiving an MS diagnosis, feel and act as if they already lost the ability to live a normal life. By introducing the concept of resilience, the ability to survive and succeed despite hardship and adversity and telling the story of patients who thrived despite having MS, this book can improve the lives of patients who live with a chronic and challenging neurological disease."

—Anonymous Academic Reviewer

"Dr. Beaber's primary goal is to demonstrate to those living with multiple sclerosis or any significant life stressors/struggles that the character trait of resilience can have a tremendous positive impact on one's happiness and even functional status in the face of adversity. His corollary goal is to demonstrate that while some people seem to be innately resilient, this a trait that to a large degree can be taught and incorporated into one's approach to living with whatever struggles one may face. The author has done a phenomenal amount of research on the topic of resilience. He has also consulted and interviewed other experts in the field to get their insights and opinions on the topics presented."

—Anonymous Academic Reviewer

"The work is clearly laid out, easy to follow, and the chapters flow logically from one to another. The case reports are all compelling and provide strong examples of how resilience plays a pivotal role in helping individuals transcend the limitations of a disease like MS."

—Anonymous Academic Reviewer

To my wife, Elana

CONTENTS

FOREWORD

by Sky-Ellen Beaber Ph.D.

ALL OF US, at some point in our life, will face circumstances that challenge us. Some of these are acute situational stressors, such as the loss of a job, death of a family member, or perhaps loss of a romantic partnership. Other forms of adversity are more insidious and pervasive.

In this book, Dr. Beaber presents compelling stories, the individual experiences of his patients coping with a chronic and progressive illness, multiple sclerosis. He lays forth these biographies, along with data and research on psychological resilience and coping strategies. While many of us will not face a diagnosis of MS in this lifetime, we are all certain to encounter pain, suffering, and the unavoidable realization that much in this world is unfair, difficult, and often not what we expected. Learning more about ways we can cope when life throws us curveballs is one way of feeling some sense of agency in a world with many factors outside our control.

I remind myself that these stories are a particular subset of patients—those with health insurance. These stories are people with access to Dr. Beaber's care, expertise, and knowledge. Whenever we read a narrative, we might also ask ourselves, "Whose story or experience am I reading? What other stories are not being told?"

As a psychologist, I also see a very specific subset of individuals in suffering, patients who either have health insurance or the means to pay for therapy out of pocket. In this day and age with rising costs, health care and mental health care have become inaccessible to many. Keeping this in mind, I invite you to read the following examples, remembering that a multiplicity of factors influence our response to stress, our reaction to suffering, and our ability to tolerate loss. To have the fullest understanding of an individual's circumstance and response, we must take into account the wider societal context.

How do we come to understand and cope with loss? This is the question Dr. Beaber seeks to answer through his exploration. These stories center around loss. In the most narrow and reductionist definition, loss manifests in a medical illness like MS as losing different bodily functions. However, this is just one piece of the story. Loss may encompass loss of autonomy, privacy, relationships, parts of identity, or certain hopes and dreams for the future. Only each individual can answer what is lost for them. Loss is unavoidable, and some losses are easier to tolerate or accept than others. To understand the reality of living with an illness, one that is chronic and potentially progressive, we must understand what it means to face loss and grief. We must understand the discomfort that comes with accepting that we rarely know how things will unfold, that much is unknowable and uncertain in life. These stories are about loss, but they are also about hope, perseverance, endurance, acceptance and compassion.

As I work in the mental health field and not the medical field, I am most able to speak to resilience from my experience using CBT (Cognitive Behavioral Therapy) and ACT (Acceptance and Commitment Therapy) as approaches to care. As a cognitive behavioral therapist, I focus on my patient's thoughts, as our thoughts can impact our moods and behaviors. An example of this is the way many people respond to a break up, perhaps one of the most common examples of loss that we encounter. When a relationship ends, people may say to themselves, "This is terrible; I'm so lonely and upset; I can't stand it!" Their narrative may be, "I'll never find love again; I will always be alone, and life just isn't worth living." This train of thinking contains many cognitive distortions, catastrophizing, fortune telling (predicting the future), along with an underestimation of one's ability to cope. Anyone repeating these distressing statements to themselves is likely to feel hopeless. Often, our thoughts are so automatic and move so quickly we don't even notice what it is we are saying to ourselves. When I meet with patients, I encourage them to pay close attention to their thoughts, to really slow down and notice what it is they say to themselves. A mindfulness practice allows a person to observe their own cognitive patterns. We have the agency, once we identify these stories, to start to change how we relate to them. The person who says to themselves the negative statements above is at much greater risk of depression and self-harm.

In Miguel's story (Chapter 8), there is a point where he reflects on the way his thinking shifts:

In my head, I was asking, 'How can you be happy with all of this happening?' What else are you to be? Sad and shitty for the rest of your life or just happy because you woke up today? Let's go with happy.

This quote reflects a pivotal point in Miguel's journey, where he starts to recognize he has choices in how he relates to his situation.

The ACT theoretical lens reminds us we are all trying to live lives full of value and meaning. Understanding one's values can provide guidance in moments where we face hardship or need to make difficult decisions. Perhaps we can't always live out our values in the ideal way we would like to, but we may still have options. Dr. James Bhat (Chapter 4) strikes me in that he highly values his work. Dr. Bhat came up with some creative solutions to continue to practice psychiatry due to his value of work, such as hiring a driver for his commute and using a baby monitor to speak to patients in the waiting room. This is one example of how one may take a step to live out important values, even in the face of changing circumstances and ability.

Another example of this is Martha Collins (Chapter 10). Martha's story speaks of her deeply held values around being a parent and having a family. Faith and service are also central to her values and life story.

Woven throughout the book are other examples of individuals continuing to pursue their values. The interview with Miguel Hernandez shows his values of love, relationships, work, learning, and inner strength. Miguel speaks positively about his parents for their hard work and perseverance, and his own continuous striving for education and job opportunities reflects his internalization of these values. Sandra Orozco's story (Chapter 6) centers on her values of service, justice, and independence.

Medical professionals are not trained, as mental health professionals are, to help clients identify their thoughts and work on reframing them or relating to them differently. Having access to these tools can make a significant difference in a client's experience of receiving a medical diagnosis. It is important not to accept all of our thoughts as facts. We have all kinds of thoughts, some insightful and transformative, and some that are exaggerations and fears rather than facts. Learning to discern the difference between these thoughts can have a positive impact on one's experience. Additionally, we can continue to live in value-congruent ways while having distressing thoughts by not allowing them to take us off our path. Dr. Beaber presents a thorough review of these tools to assist both patients and professionals.

When my brother first told to me he planned to write this book, we discussed what topics might be helpful to include and what I might contribute. I shared my experience of studying mindfulness both professionally and personally and the ways I have integrated it into my practice. My first experience with mindfulness was a deep dive into a seven-day meditation retreat. The retreat included multiple "sits" per day, as well as yoga, a moving mindfulness practice. This week was transformative for me, as I felt my nervous system really settle in a way it never had before. Fortunately, you do not need a seven-day retreat to achieve the benefits of mindfulness (although it certainly is a beneficial experience!) We can take mindful pauses throughout our day and build a practice in as little as a few minutes a day. Teaching clients mindfulness skills can be a very powerful way to help people to sit with, observe, and accept "what is." Although the impact of my own retreat experience was relaxing, mindfulness does not always result in feeling "good." In fact, the intention of mindfulness is not to change our current state—but to fully experience and observe what is. Often, when we are struggling to live out one of our values, the experience is far from relaxing and pleasant. We must accept the whole range of emotions and thoughts that coincides with living a meaningful life.

My second experience was a five-day retreat with Dr. Kristin Neff. Dr. Beaber details some of Dr. Neff's teachings on self-compassion in Chapter 9. This retreat, not unlike the first, transformed my relationship to myself and to my work. In my years of practice, one ongoing theme I observe is that clients are often *very hard* on themselves. When we are already suffering, berating ourselves only leads to additional suffering. Unfortunately, many of us believe that self-blame and self-critique will lead to us making progress towards our goals. However, it is quite the opposite. In her book, Dr. Neff details the research that shows the way the "brain on shame" negatively impacts our motivation to look at the very areas where we need to grow. If we can be kind to ourselves, loving, forgiving, and compassionate, our experience of suffering attenuates. This is an invaluable coping strategy for all of us, whether we are facing a chronic illness, or another stressor.

While there is currently no "cure" for MS, the ideas in this book give us some framework for coping and thriving. The review of the literature on psychological resilience, mindfulness, Ho'oponopono, logotherapy, etc. provides us with strategies on how to relate to and contend with the experience of impermanence and suffering. In these personal narratives, we gain some insight into the moments we have choice, and in those choices lies our freedom.

CHAPTER 1:
MULTIPLE SCLEROSIS

"I want America to know that you can still have
a full, exciting, and productive life even if you or your loved
one is battling a debilitating, chronic disease such as MS."
—Michaele Salahi

My head was spinning. I was in severe pain. On a scale of one to ten, it was a twenty. I couldn't even turn my head to the left because I was in such pain. I had paralysis of my right face. My throat had closed down, and I could not eat. I had peripheral blindness of both eyes. I felt like I was dying. I lost faith. I lost hope. I lost my career as a healthcare professional. I was slowly going into a state of depression, and I felt worthless to society. I went to my nephew Jonathan when he was seven days old, and I said to him, "I'm not going to be around. I'm going to be a little angel watching over you."

THESE ARE THE words of Sandra Orozco, a then thirty-eight-year-old hospital administrator. She was an energetic and ambitious young woman with the world as her oyster, but the attack on January 19th, 1993 left her scared and hopeless. The mysterious illness started with a vague imbalance followed by vertigo, blackouts, and a shutdown of half the functions of her nervous system. Perhaps worst of all was the widespread pain—burning, tingling, sharp, stinging—like a blanket of hot coals with electric shocks striking stochastically. It was not just her body that failed her but her self-confidence and her entire support system. When you are ill and no one knows why, sometimes people assume that it is self-inflicted or you just are not trying hard enough. Even those who love us prefer to "blame the victim" rather than acknowledge that life can be arbitrary, cruel, and tragic. Sandra's remembrance of her childhood is not atypical of the family interactions that haunt children with mystifying symptoms.

"You're fat. You're ugly. Your teeth are bad…no man's gonna want you. You're no good for nobody." My mom said that. If I would say something, she would hit me. I was crying. I would not take a bath. I didn't care about myself or my acquaintances. I didn't want to go out. I didn't want to eat.

These sound like the words of a woman battered, beaten, and crushed by adversity, but when I met Sandra in 2016, she had become one of the strongest and most inspirational people I have ever known. It was not because of a fortuitous recovery or miracle cure. On the contrary, she has used a wheelchair for years and is plagued by a myriad of symptoms both conspicuous and invisible. She has battled depression, family conflict, and a host of personal demons. However, everyone she meets can see something which is quite profound: An infectious smile, an appreciation for little things, a philanthropic purpose, and a passion for life. She is optimistic, personable, and productive. She reoriented her organizational and leadership talents towards a life of political activism and has become a pillar of strength in her community. She has meaningful social relationships, and she wakes up every morning with something to do. Over the years, she has won awards, shaped the local political landscape, and even took part in uncovering the infamous City of Bell scandal in 2010.

Sandra is just one of the amazing people I have met over the years. The forthcoming chapters will elucidate their inspirational stories, returning to Sandra in Chapter Six. These narratives unveil the hidden powers of psychological resilience that can salvage a life plagued by a terrifying illness. They remind us of a truism. Life might be described as a war between human-kind and disease, accidents, homicide, and aging. That war is punctuated by smaller battles and skirmishes modern medicine graciously allows us to win. Alas, while we may win some battles, our shared destiny is to lose the war. Accordingly, the measure of any person cannot be victory but only the dignity with which he or she conducts the struggle. Our defining character can only be our psychological resilience. I hope these stories of resilience will be instructive, heartwarming, and inspiring.

INTRODUCTION

As a clinical neurologist, I have the unique experience of spending a significant amount of time with people who have physical limitations. I specialize in treating multiple sclerosis (MS) and other immunological diseases of the nervous system. MS affects nearly one million Americans[1] and has a profound physical and emotional impact on their lives. However, even when people develop serious disabilities from the disease, they often find a way to thrive and not just survive.

You may ask, "Why write a book exploring the resilient qualities of individuals with MS?" Three reasons: First, I think they can provide us life lessons we can all benefit from, whether or not we suffer from a particular disease. Second, by drawing attention to their resilient qualities, I am hoping to ensure that they, and others with significant health conditions, come to see themselves in this light as well. And third, I want those not intimately involved in the MS community to learn more about the condition and have a taste of what it is like to live with a disability.

MS is a fascinating disease. A detailed description of the extensive scientific knowledge on this topic is beyond the scope of this work, but I will give you an overview to provide some context. Multiple sclerosis is named after areas of scar-like tissue, known as sclerotic plaques, in the brain, spinal cord, and optic nerves of affected patients. MS damages the myelin, a fatty sheath that normally protects the nerve fibers. The myelin aids in the speedy and efficient communication between cells within the nervous system. A schematic of a normal nerve fiber with surrounding myelin is shown in Figure 1.

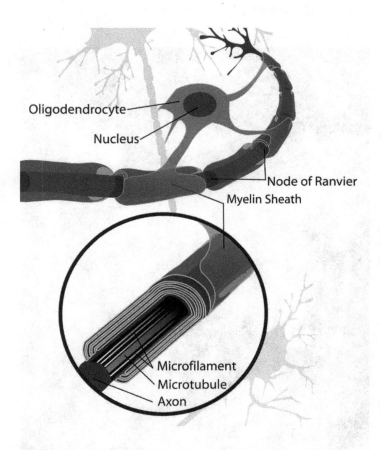

Figure 1. A myelin-covered nerve fiber reminds us of an electrical wire with insulation. The oligodendrocytes are supportive cells that produce myelin in the central nervous system. Source of graphic: Wikimedia Commons.

Magnetic resonance imaging (MRI) scans of the nervous system in patients with MS often reveal impressive macrostructural changes. Such changes are shown in the image below (Figure 2). Compare this to a normal MRI (Figure 3).

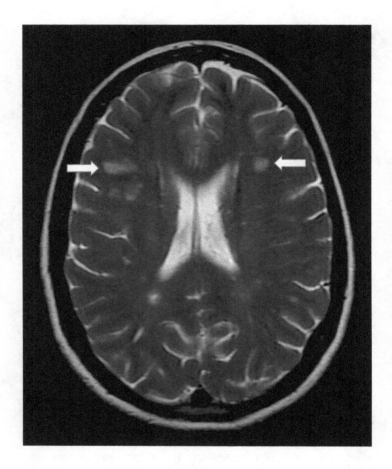

Figure 2. An MRI showing abnormal plaques in the white matter typical of multiple sclerosis (some of which are noted by arrows). Source of graphic: Wikimedia Commons.

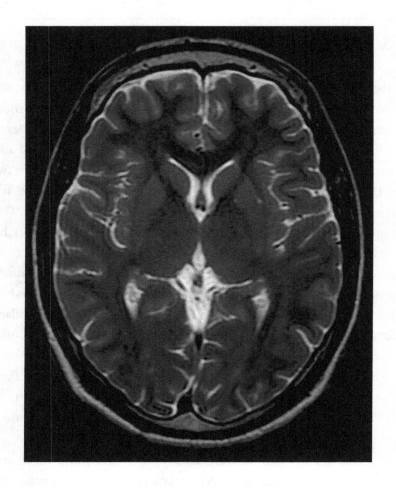

Figure 3. A normal MRI of the brain (T2 axial sequence).
Source of graphic: Wikimedia Commons.

The potential ramifications of MS are endless, because almost
everything about who we are and what we do is a manifestation
of the central nervous system. This includes our senses, memories,
abilities, personalities, tendencies, and even morals. For more on the
philosophical significance of the nervous system, see **Appendix D**

MS BASICS

At the outset, it is helpful to have a sense of the brain and its attached nervous system. The nervous system is, at its core, the most elegant and robust communication system in the known universe. It is composed of billions of cells (neurons) that chatter back and forth among themselves, conversing with all the senses and muscles that control dexterity and ambulation. It is responsible for hearing, speech, interpreting speech, and fashioning responses. The brain learns by storing information, and it regulates activities by retrieving information, implementing plans, and sending orders to muscles. Through the optic nerves, the brain obtains visual information from the environment. Much of the brain is dedicated to integration, correspondence between various parts, and secondary processing. Hence, the brain, with its neurons, is the organ of communication within the body. Any disease or pathology that impedes, retards, or garbles this communication process results in a wide array of impairments. MS is just one of numerous diseases that interfere with our internal communication apparatus, and it has its own unique tendencies and peculiarities.

MS has two major clinical presentations: a relapsing form and a progressive form. Relapsing MS is marked by the dramatic development of neurological symptoms, such as vision loss, vertigo, numbness or weakness, followed by relative quiescence. The attacks of symptoms are called "relapses," and the intervening periods are called "remissions." Progressive MS, on the other hand, causes a more continuous and insidious decline in neurological function, often manifesting with gait impairment or cognitive dysfunction. This steady worsening is known as "progression." Relapsing MS is more common in younger individuals, and progressive MS is more common in older individuals. The two forms can overlap, and relapsing MS can transition into progressive MS. Progressive MS has a more negative connotation because it is often associated with greater disability than relapsing MS.

Relapsing MS appears to be sparked primarily by abnormal inflammation, and white blood cells invade the central nervous system, causing injury. Progressive MS appears to be at least partly degenerative and can resemble Alzheimer's disease or Parkinson's disease. The cause of MS is unknown, but evidence suggests that the immune system becomes dysregulated and attacks the body's own tissues, analogous to autoimmune diseases such as lupus or rheumatoid arthritis. Various risk factors for MS have been identified. These include living far from the equator, having low blood levels of vitamin D, having a history of mononucleosis (the "kissing disease," which causes fatigue), smoking, being born in May, and having a family history of the disease. There is also evidence that MS is more common in developed countries, suggesting that Western diet, lack of sunlight, and modern hygiene play a role. However, the underlying cause of MS is unknown.

No one can predict with any reasonable accuracy who will develop MS, so it could happen to anyone. I have patients who are physicians, scientologists, long-term vegans, paleo-diet fanatics, triathletes, and marathon runners. Many celebrities have MS including the following:

- Josh Harding—former professional hockey goalie for the Minnesota Wild
- Chris Wright—professional basketball player
- Montel Williams—talk show host
- Trevor Bayne—NASCAR driver and former Daytona 500 winner
- Jack Osbourne—TV star
- Ann Romney—wife of Mitt Romney, former Massachusetts governor and presidential candidate
- Michaele Salahi—from The Real Housewives of DC

- Neil Cavuto—Fox news anchor
- Clay Walker—country music star
- Alan and David Osmond—from the famous Osmond family (David Osmond is well known in the MS community)
- Annette Funicello (1942-2013)—former Disney Mouseketeer and actor
- Richard Pryor (1940-2005)—comedian
- Richard Cohen—journalist
- Clive Burr—drummer for the band Iron Maiden
- Teri Garr—comedian and actor
- Tamia Hill—R&B singer, actress (also the wife of former pro basketball player Grant Hill)

A CLINICAL DESCRIPTION OF MS

One interesting aspect of the disease is the incredible variability in its severity. Some individuals are incidentally found at autopsy to have brain lesions highly typical of MS despite never reporting symptoms during their lifetime. Others clearly have clinical MS, but they recover quickly from relapses, never develop progressive MS, and live a long, healthy life, with or without treatment. Still others have moderate problems with varying degrees of severity. Finally, an unlucky few have very aggressive or even fatal variants of MS. I have 70-year-old MS patients with minimal problems who eat a poor diet, do not exercise, and smoke cigarettes. Often, these people have more non–MS-related health problems than MS-related health problems. I have twenty-one-year-old healthy and fit patients with serious impairments. No one can consistently prognosticate the course of MS at the time of diagnosis—a terrifying thought if you are a healthy 20-year-old with a mild first attack.

MS can also cause a lot of invisible and subjective symptoms. Fatigue, heat sensitivity, poor concentration, cognitive fogging, unusual sensations, and neuropathic pain are common. These symptoms are often more significant to people with MS than conspicuous findings such as vision loss or weakness. I have patients who walk normally but are on disability because of these symptoms, and I have patients in wheelchairs who work sixty hours a week. Disability is often imperceptible and individual. The list of potential MS symptoms is so long that almost anyone could be convinced they have the condition. Have you ever had any of the following symptoms: blurry vision, double vision, pain, muscle spasms, tightening around the abdomen or chest, numbness, tingling, dizziness, balance difficulty, constipation, loose stools, erectile dysfunction, frequent urination, waking up at night to urinate, "brain fog," poor concentration, fatigue, speech difficulty, disorganization, depression, anxiety, or heat intolerance? It would be truly remarkable for someone to have no symptoms associated with MS whatsoever. I routinely do consultations for people who are wrongly convinced that they have MS after researching the condition online.

Many of my patients look completely normal to a layperson, and they suffer silently. Often, people do not tell their friends, coworkers, or bosses they have a disease. I have had patients who do not even tell their significant others—even after several years and even if they are married. Vision loss, numbness, fatigue, mild cognitive dysfunction, and pain can be difficult for a casual observer to discern. Even a detailed neurological examination and an MRI scan can only tell you so much. In my field, the best piece of diagnostic equipment is the ear.

TREATMENTS

The past twenty-five years have seen significant advances in the medical treatment of MS. Although reports of the condition date back hundreds of years, the availability of MRI starting around

1980 has made a big difference in diagnosis. The first pharmaceutical drug to treat MS (Betaseron©) was approved by the Food and Drug Administration (FDA) in 1993, and at the time of this writing, the FDA has approved seventeen drugs for MS. Some of these are highly effective at reducing new MRI lesions and preventing clinical attacks, and the trend is toward more targeted treatments with fewer systemic side effects. Various remedies are available to help with the symptoms of MS including medications for neuropathic pain and specialized mobility devices. There are also non-standard treatments, such as specialized diets and other alternative therapies. If you search "multiple sclerosis" in the US National Library of Medicine–National Institutes of Health (PubMed), you will find over 75,000 articles. MS research receives funding from various sources, including the National Institutes of Health, the National Multiple Sclerosis Society (a charitable organization), private donors, and pharmaceutical companies.

I am very optimistic about the long-term prospects of improving treatment or even curing MS. Now is a better time than ever to be diagnosed, and in thirty years what we do now will seem archaic and brutish. Much of modern MS research looks at finding the cause of MS and learning how to address the degenerative aspects of the disease. Can we offer neuroprotective treatments that will prevent a slow decline in function in our patients with progressive MS? Can we learn to regrow neural tissue to improve function even in those with longstanding disabilities associated with the loss of neurons and axons? Until then, millions of people are waiting impatiently with hope, apprehension, or even anger.

When you watch the news, you get the impression a medical breakthrough or miracle cure is discovered every day. However, when you have a specific disease, most medical advances do not apply to your situation, so progress seems much slower. Journalists tend to exaggerate the significance of health news, and this leads to a lot of disappointment and frustration. We already have a hundred cures for MS; they just do not work—at least not for everyone. A google search for "multiple sclerosis" will dispel any doubt that MS patients are constantly besieged with "fake" news of an imminent cure. Clearly, hope predicated on unrealistic expectations is a double-edged sword.

RESILIENCE

From time to time, I think about what would happen to me if I became disabled. Would I be bitter and hateful? Would I feel cursed as though fate had turned against me? Would I be consumed by my illness, allowing it to take over my life and to define me as a person? When asked to characterize me, would a friend start by saying "Brandon has disease X"? Or would he start by talking about my personality, actions, hopes, and dreams? I imagine it would be extremely difficult to adjust to having a disease such as MS, particularly if I had significant disabilities. My life is so dependent on my being physically fit, energetic, emotionally sound, and mentally sharp. This is because I work nights and weekends, exercise regularly, and attend to my family, friends, and hobbies. I am constantly on the go, meeting immediate obligations and planning for the future. Even mild problems would force me to completely revamp my lifestyle.

This book is not about MS itself. Rather, it focuses on how people react to the disease and rebuild their lives in the face of adversity. In particular, I will tell five stories about exceptional individuals with MS who achieve great things and have a high quality of life despite significant hardship. These patients shocked me with their resilience, and they inspired me to write this book. They include a neurologist, a psychiatrist, a political activist, a young blind man, and a woman with advanced MS. Except for Sandra Orozco, the political activist, I have changed their names and institutional affiliations for professional privacy. They all have very different backgrounds and problems, and they each appear to approach MS in their own unique way. We will explore their childhood, their history of MS, their achievements, and the things they do to improve their lives and to adapt to the disease. What can we learn from these amazing people? What makes them different? Are there underlying commonalities we can emulate? Are they simply lucky, or is their ability to overcome MS the result of specific characteristics or proactive behavior? Can they teach us how to face the conflicts we are all destined to experience?

I am confident it is actually possible for people with MS to feel stronger and more resilient than they felt before receiving the diagnosis. I have seen this many times, and there is often a striking evolution from the initial reaction to the disease. At the onset, many are anticipating the worst, overwhelmed by ruminating fears, or even clinically depressed.

For those who would later feel stronger and more resilient than before their diagnosis, their experience is consistent with what clinical researchers Richard Tedeschi, Ph.D. and Lawrence Calhoun, Ph.D. refer to as "posttraumatic growth." Their studies reveal potential growth in the following five general areas following major life crises: 1) Increased awareness of new opportunities and new possibilities; 2) Stronger personal relationships and stronger emotional connections to others who suffer; 3) Greater awareness of personal strength despite also being more aware of vulnerability to traumatic events beyond one's control; 4) Valuing life more than before and growing more appreciative of things that previously might have been taken for granted; and 5) Experiencing a deeper spiritual life, sometimes also resulting in a change in one's belief system. While Tedeschi and Calhoun[2,3] remind us that posttraumatic growth should not be construed as the opposite of posttraumatic stress, research shows it is conceivable, albeit not universal, that from intense pain and distress can also come growth[4].

As we examine these five fascinating stories, you will note how each of their life journeys reflect growth in several of these areas. We will also look more deeply into the science, psychology, and practical development of resilience. Extensive research has shown it can have a profound impact on our lives, and whether or not we have MS, we are certain to have our resilience tested many times. Psychologists have also taken an interest in resilience, and we will discuss the input from various schools of thought. Later on, we will look into pragmatic techniques, including the philosophy of Ho'oponopono and the practice of mindfulness meditation. Each story and each concept gives us some wisdom we need to approach conflict in life.

"All men are brave," Emerson once wrote, "But heroes are brave five minutes longer." Some of the most resilient people we will ever have the pleasure of meeting have to work very hard just to make it through a normal day. As such, I hope to tell these stories candidly, showing not just the glamor of success but also the very real and painful struggles people have with MS. All five of my subjects had a rocky road in life, and this makes their accomplishments that much more spectacular. We will begin with my colleague in neurology, Dr. Emily Spitz. Many people in my field have influenced the way I think about my career, but she is one of the few who has truly changed the way I think about life.

CHAPTER ONE REFERENCES

1. Culpepper WJ, Marrie RA, Langer-Gould A, et al. Validation of an algorithm for identifying MS cases in administrative health claims databases. Neurology March 05, 2019;92 (10).
2. Tedeschi RG, Cann A, Taku K, Senol-Durak E, Calhoun LG. The Posttraumatic Growth Inventory: A Revision Integrating Existential and Spiritual Change. J Trauma Stress. 2017 Feb;30(1):11-18.
3. Cann A, Calhoun LG, Tedeschi RG, Taku K, Vishnevsky T, Triplett KN, Danhauer SC. A short form of the Posttraumatic Growth Inventory. Anxiety Stress Coping. 2010;23(2):127-37
4. *Katz M. Children Who Fail at School But Succeed at Life: Lessons from Lives Well-Lived. W.W. Norton & Company April 11, 2016.*

CHAPTER 2:
DR. EMILY SPITZ

"You have brains in your head. You have feet in your shoes. You can steer yourself any direction you choose. You're on your own. And you know what you know. And YOU are the one who'll decide where to go..."
— Dr. Seuss, *Oh, The Places You'll Go!*

I WORKED WITH DR. Spitz for many years, and I have grown to know her well. When I was a senior resident, she was an internal medicine intern at the same institution. When I was a fellow doing subspecialty training, she was a resident in my neurology department. I later became an attending physician, and I acted as her supervisor at times, rounding with her in the hospital and mentoring her in clinic. I knew she had MS from the start, and she was treated by a close colleague and mentor of mine. I was even personally involved in her care as you will soon see. Emily is not disabled. If you saw her, you would not know that she has MS, but her resilience is truly admirable. I know this because I found internship and residency to be challenging enough without MS, and I witnessed firsthand some of what she had to fight through. This chapter describes her past, her history of MS, and her unusual experience as a neurologist with MS.

Emily was born in Boulder Creek, a small mountain town near Santa Cruz, California. Her parents were free-flowing non-traditional "hippies" with a small family business. Before she was born, her parents lived on a boat, and they sold doors, windows, stained glass, and other handmade products, transporting things ashore in a small dinghy. When her mother became pregnant, they decided they wanted to raise Emily in a more traditional setting. Hence, they moved back to her mother's hometown and rented a house from Emily's maternal grandfather.

> It was a pretty small house—nothing special. There was an acre and a quarter of land, and my parents believed strongly that we should have lots of outdoor space and outdoor time. We had chickens and peacocks; we raised our own eggs; we had our own garden. I have a brother two-and-a-half years younger than me, and when I was growing up, my elementary school years were pretty traditional. My parents were very supportive. My mom was a strong believer that you shouldn't charge

more money than is absolutely justified, so there was never a lot of money lying around.

To compound the financial problems, Emily's father has a disability from a motorcycle accident which occurred when he was twenty-two. The accident damaged his brachial plexus, a cluster of nerves connecting the spine to the arm. This left him with only minimal movement in his dominant arm which now hangs uselessly with tightened spastic muscles. Although he has had this problem since before Emily was born, she still remembers him crafting custom doors by hand and lifting heavy objects. It was never a major concern, and it is only a passing detail of childhood by her account.

Her early upbringing was generally without significant drama, but tension later developed because of her mother's infidelity.

When I was a teenager, my mom had an affair, and it ended up causing a fair amount of conflict in my family because I knew about it. My dad wanted to stay with my mom for the children's sake. I was the advocate for my dad. I remember I had a conversation with my mom, and I was like, "Mom, you need to stop this; don't you realize what this is doing?" But she was like, "It makes me happy." I think I was like, "Well, it's her or us." It's a weird conversation to have as the kid, right? I've always been a little bit of the adult in my family. They ended up, after about a year, getting a divorce, and my brother and I moved with my dad a couple of miles down the street while my mom stayed in the same house where we grew up. Still, my parents were both very supportive and would do anything for us.

From the beginning, Emily was a good student, and she was attracted to science and math. She had no exposure to the field of medicine, but she wanted to be a doctor as early as the 3rd grade, and this gave her a goal to work towards. She did well in high school, and she eventually went to UC Davis which was close to home yet far enough away that her parents would not drop in on her too often. However, at age seventeen before she left for college, she experienced what was in hindsight her first multiple sclerosis attack. In her description, she uses the term "ataxia" which refers to clumsiness of gait.

It was probably late winter or early spring. It was a sunny day, and I developed a little bit of ataxia and weakness; I don't remember which side it was on. We had an outdoor campus, and my hip just kept bumping against the rail as I was walking. I was just like, "Why can't I walk?"

I didn't think much of it, and to get around, I just had to have someone walk with me so I wouldn't bump into things. I could walk independently, but I would bump into things along the way. At the time, I was on the basketball team. I was never very good, but I was on the team. I remember very clearly we had a game. I was an assistant guard, and I would dribble the ball and what not. I could jog, but I was slower than I normally was. I couldn't coordinate doing multiple things. I remember very clearly: I was in a game, and I caught the ball. I thought to myself, "Work the ball up the court," and I couldn't coordinate in my mind dribbling the ball and running at the same time. I attempted to, and I ended up fumbling the ball and falling down.

She never even saw a doctor as mainstream medicine was simply not part of the family culture. They just took herbal remedies and other traditional therapies. Her father encouraged her to rest in a calm and optimistic tone, and she improved within days. As a neurologist, she retrospectively thinks it odd her parents did not make a big deal about the episode, but I have heard similar stories a thousand times. MS relapses can lead to all sorts of alternative explanations such as natural clumsiness, orthopedic injuries, or even aging. People can have five or six attacks before they are diagnosed.

After she recovered, Emily went on with her life, graduated high school, and left for UC Davis. She made many new friends, and she also dated the man who would later become her husband. Her initial research experience was in cardiology, and she originally had ambitions of being an internist. She later took a course in neurobiology and ended up majoring in the combined field of neurobiology, physiology, and behavior. Still, she did not think about a career in neurology until she was diagnosed with MS.

The next attack happened during her second year in college about a month before her twenty-first birthday. She came out of a physics class and got on her bicycle to ride home when she realized a subtle lack of coordination. She could not steady herself enough to ride, and she fell off the bike. Knowing something was wrong, she walked over to the student health center. The staff performed routine urine and blood tests and told her to "sleep it off" as though she were an inebriated sorority sister.

The next morning, I woke up, and I went to get out of bed. I couldn't walk, and I stumbled into my closet. I had to call a friend, and I said, "I need to go back to the student health center."

Her legs were weak and clumsy, and she returned to student health, demanding they take her seriously. Luckily, a general practitioner advocated for her and called a local tertiary care center to arrange an MRI. They planned an outpatient MRI within a few weeks and send her home to wait. You would think she would be terrified and anxious, wondering what strange paralytic illness could cause the symptoms, but she was contented by having a plan in place and went home to be cared for by her roommate and friends.

I was in bed for a couple of days, and my friends helped me and brought me food. During that time, I developed double vision which made reading, studying, and watching TV rather difficult because everything made me nauseous. I don't think I was scared at all which is a little bit strange. In hindsight, I kind of look at it and go, "What was I thinking?" I was scared that things wouldn't get better, but I don't think I was really scared because it got better before, so why wouldn't it get better again? It did get better, and in a couple of days, my dad came and picked me up. I think I said something to the extent of, "Dad, I need help walking," and he said "Oh, you'll walk it off," and he made me go on a walk around the block. I left having a lot of difficulty, leaning on him a bit, and when I came back, I was walking nearly independently. He said, "You can do it; you can do it." So, I did it.

She was home for the weekend but went back to class the next Monday. Emily was not the type to miss a lot of school, and during her time off, she was more bored than fearful.

I remember being bored, and I remember being frustrated because of my vision during the attack. What else are you supposed to do? You can't read; you can't walk; you can't watch TV. What do you do?

She had the MRI scan and made a follow up appointment with a physician to review the results, and the doctor made the diagnosis confidently without the need for a spinal tap. He sat down lower than eye level and spoke in a slow and calming tone: "I am very sorry to tell you this, but you have a disorder that's called multiple sclerosis."

I think I just nodded, and I said, "Okay." I don't think I knew what that meant. I just said, "Okay; what do I do next?" "We're going to send you to a neurologist, and we're going to get you on medication," and I said, "Okay."

By this time, she had fully recovered. Often, people with MS receive steroids such as methylprednisolone through an IV to speed rehabilitation, but many attacks improve spontaneously. She went home and googled "multiple sclerosis." Often, this will lead to a lot of fear and confusion, but Emily learned a lot of basic information about the condition in a short period, and this made her feel more confident and grounded. She followed up with a neurologist who recommended she start Avonex©, a once a week intramuscular injection which decreases MS relapses and accumulation of MS plaques on MRI. She practiced the injections on an orange, stabbing the poor orange "to death" until she mastered the technique. The student health pharmaceutical plan only covered six weeks of the very expensive medication, but luckily, her father had a new job with full benefits, and he was able to add Emily onto his insurance plan.

As doctors, we prescribe medications with the flick of a pen or the click of a mouse, but the actual logistics can be somewhat more arduous. It took Emily several weeks to acquire the medication, and she ended up doing her first injection with the help of a friend at two o'clock in the morning. Sticking a needle in your own thigh is harder than you think, and I would know since I once took Avonex© myself on a whim. Emily was terrified to give herself the shot, but she didn't want to "look like a wuss," so she plunged in the needle with authority. She had horrible muscle aches and local soreness as side effects, and she drove home to sleep it off. Soon after this, she visited her boyfriend and took Avonex© before going to sleep. Her rigors were so significant that he kept waking up, thinking she was in the "throes of dying." In reality, she slept through it, oblivious to what was going on.

> He tells these stories of the day I took the medicine and almost died, and I'm like, "It was the day I was sleeping; calm down."

Side effects are an idiosyncratic thing. I have tried various MS drugs over the years just to experience them. I felt fine when I took Avonex© and did an hour of hill sprints immediately afterwards. For many, however, the severe secondary effects can make continuing the medication impractical. With these potent reactions and a $50,000-per-year price tag, you would think Avonex© is a bona fide MS cure. Unfortunately, the results from clinical trials are marginal at best[1, 2], and pharmaceutical companies have been widely criticized[3, 4].

Although taking prescription pharmaceuticals for human disease has become a well-established part of American culture, some people find that taking a medication can have a detrimental psychological effect as it constantly reminds them they are a "sick" person. Besides causing side effects, the daily regimen forces you to think about the disease, and this often exacerbates some otherwise subtle symptoms. Emily did not experience this negative psychology and did not seriously consider the long-term consequences of MS until much later. After all, her attacks were brief, and she recovered without treatment. At this point, it would be hard to call her resilient because her nonchalance was more due to naiveté than character strength.

At the time of diagnosis, Emily was a sophomore in college. She was on the pre-med track, studying hard and doing research on the side. Nonetheless, she found the time to interact with the MS community at large. She learned more about the disease, took part in MS fundraisers, and spoke at sorority houses to spread awareness. MS is the most common disabling condition amongst young women, but many people have never even heard of it or are only vaguely familiar with it. She collected small donations in twenty-dollar increments for National MS Society events, often raising over $1,000. She was comfortable disclosing her diagnosis and remembers how surprised her fellow students were to see how good she looked.

Her insurance changed again, forcing her into the care of another neurologist, but she remained on the same treatment. She had MS relapses roughly annually, but they were relatively mild, and at worst, she would receive a few days of IV steroids. During these episodes, she would have numbness of the limbs or slight weakness, but she never lost any significant function. She eventually graduated from college and went to medical school, and she changed physicians once again. Avonex© did not seem to be particularly effective for Emily as the typical placebo-treated patient in modern clinical trials has about one relapse per two years, half the rate that Emily had while on treatment. She also tolerated the drug poorly, continuing to have muscle aches and flu-like symptoms with every shot and requiring high doses of analgesics. Despite this, she stayed the course because she was doing well overall and perceived a lack of better options.

Medical school has a way of turning us all into hypochondriacs, and Emily fell victim to this as she learned more about the nature of neurological disease.

I think finally at that point I started understanding, "Oh…wait; this isn't a disorder you always get better from." That's the first time I put two and two together and realized I could end up severely disabled.

Because of this, Emily became more vigilant, and after several relapses, she switched her MS treatment to natalizumab (Tysabri©). Tysabri© is a potent monthly infusion therapy with a small but real risk of a serious viral infection of the brain called PML (progressive multifocal leukoencephalopathy). She stabilized nicely for a brief period, but blood tests revealed that Tysabri© was injuring her liver, so she switched to an oral medication called fingolimod (Gilenya©). Gilenya© is generally well tolerated, but it has a temporary effect of causing bradycardia, a slow heart rate. Emily had to undergo a six-hour observation to make sure she did not develop symptoms related to bradycardia or an abnormal heart rhythm.

I took my books and sat there, and I got down to a heart rate in the upper thirties. The poor girl who was my nurse would look at the monitor every time she would walk past. My boyfriend at the time was there, and I was chatting with him. Every time she would look, her face would blanch, and you could just see she was visibly scared. I think it was because my heart rate would just slow and slow and slow and slow because I was sitting there and not moving much. My blood pressure was low as well. I would get up and go to the bathroom because they had me on fluids, and every time I would get up, she would be like, *gasp*; "It's okay; I'm just going to the bathroom. I'm just going to pee." At one point, she was so nervous that she opened and drew up the atropine. "We'll just put this medication here in case you stop talking." "Okay; that's fine."

Emily never did require atropine (a medication to reverse bradycardia), and aside from a mild relapse which occurred shortly after changing to fingolimod, she was stable for the next two-and-a-half years. With no meaningful physical disability, she completed medical school without unexpected delays. Her personal experience with MS had shifted her interest from cardiology to neurology, and after many clinical rotations, four standardized licensing exams, and a slew of interviews, she was accepted to my neurology residency program. In the interim, she married her long-term boyfriend. She only remembers a single instance of any negative reaction to her diagnosis. I concealed the name of the institution from her description.

I did not disclose when I applied. I had one person who interviewed me at ***** if I remember correctly. It was a gentleman, and he was like, "Hello? How are you doing? Hi? Blah blah blah. So, I see you do a lot of work for MS, and I don't see that you have" …and the way he phrased it was like, "And my conclusion is that you have MS yourself." It was all very round about, shady, and backhanded. It wasn't really to get to a question. It was just so he could point out that, "Ha! I figured *out you have MS!" It was such a weird encounter that it tainted the rest of the interview for me. It was the last one of the day, and I liked the program until that point. I didn't rank it because of that experience...just because it didn't feel right. Beyond that, I don't think I've had anyone treat me differently. If anything, I have gotten special treatment at some visits because I'm a doctor which makes me feel a little guilty sometimes.*

As I said before, I was a senior resident when I first met Emily. She was starting an internal medicine internship, a required preliminary year before neurology residency. When the program director found out that Emily had MS, she set her up with Dr. Lyons, our MS specialist who was also my mentor. Dr. Lyons is an amazing neurologist—kind, knowledgeable, patient, and truly on the cutting edge of the field. Emily and I both hit the jackpot—Emily as a patient, and me as a young doctor in training. Meeting the right people makes all the difference, and I would probably be in a different subspecialty if it were not for her.

Emily had a great reputation as an intern. Smart, hard-working, and efficient, she is the type of person you can count on to get things done, to stay an extra hour, and to follow up on every critical detail. She is type A but not fretful or anxious, and she is calm in a crisis with ice-water flowing through her veins. She has a certain confidence about her and speaks to patients in an unwavering didactic tone that would not be questioned or doubted. She also has an intuitive pragmatic judgment that cannot be taught and is uncorrelated with book knowledge of medicine. When she became a senior resident, she was tough on the juniors and even made a new resident cry once while giving constructive feedback. Even I found her intimidating at times. She is rarely warm or smiling, but she cares deeply about the fate of her patients, becoming visibly upset when care is not coordinated ideally. She has a businesslike mentality and avoids complaint, banter, and gossip.

Despite being a diligent and studious resident, Emily never seemed to have a strong interest in the field of neuroimmunology. Perhaps it hit too close to home. Occasionally, she would have to admit some of my more severely affected patients to the hospital, and discussing these cases with her was always awkward. Seeing someone who has one's same condition but is much worse off is unnerving and reminds you of what could happen. Additionally, treating only the MS patients that get admitted to the hospital gives the false impression that MS uniformly causes harsh attacks and profound disability, whereas the outpatient clinic provides a much more optimistic and balanced view of the disease.

However, when she was a 2nd year resident, her fears were realized, and she had the worst attack of her life while covering the stroke service.

It was a brutal exacerbation. I was on stroke, and I had some subtle symptoms. The first thing I noticed was that my typing was uncoordinated. I was like, "That's a little weird. My typing is a little inaccurate." I thought, "Maybe I'm tired." It was really subtle. Later on, I was walking in my apartment, and I was doing something on my phone. I didn't make the turn, and I ran into the wall going into the kitchen. It was things you normally could do that I just couldn't quite do. I pulled the senior resident aside, and I was like, "I think I'm having a mild exacerbation, but can I just have you do a neuro-examination?" We go in a room in the ER. He did an exam and was like, "You're having ataxia; it's not terrible. You're obviously doing well enough to hide it from us. You are having it; you're not making it up."

She got one of the ER doctors to give her IV steroids.

A day or two after that, I was talking to a family, but while I was standing there, I became really imbalanced, so I had this whole conversation sort of holding onto the bed. When I went back up the stairs, I had to use the wall for guidance. I was on service with a couple of the radiology residents, and I was like, "I need one of you to assist me." I ordered my own steroids; I made my own infusion center appointment. I went, and I think I texted Dr. Lyons while I was there: "I'm having an exacerbation. I already set up my own steroids." I had one of the residents, and I refused to let him get me a wheelchair in spite of the fact that he was like, "You probably need a wheelchair." I was leaning pretty heavily on him. That's who I am; I don't like to ask for help. I let people help me, but I don't like to let things be easy.

Unfortunately, Emily continued to deteriorate, and my mentor was out of the office. I ended up visiting her in the infusion center while she was receiving her last dose of Solumedrol©. After a few pleasantries and an introduction to her husband who had driven down to visit her, I treated her as I would any other patient. I was taken aback by her condition. She could barely walk unassisted, and it was unsafe for her to try. Her legs were weak and clumsy, and she could not lift her toes on one side, so her foot dragged across the floor as she tried to move forward. Her gait was wide-based and tremulous. She was anxious, quavering in her voice, and on the verge of tears. I had never seen her like this. As a doctor, I am very accustomed to being around sick people. Perhaps, I am desensitized, but when it is a friend or a relative, I somehow lose my normal immunity, and I feel the same visceral disturbance a layperson would. I advised she be admitted to the hospital for plasmapheresis, a dialysis-like procedure which removes abnormal inflammatory antibodies from the blood stream. I also recommended that she change Gilenya© to a stronger MS treatment. Dr. Lyons later agreed over the phone.

Aside from the usual frustrations of inpatient care, her treatment went smoothly. To have plasmapheresis, she had to undergo a procedure to place a large venous catheter in the jugular vein in her neck. This was uncomfortable but tolerated, and there were no complications. She had an irritable roommate, and she once had to wait forty minutes before a nurse could help her navigate to the restroom. However, the treatment worked, and she was already improving by the time of discharge. Despite all the drama, one of her main complaints about the hospital stay was the "incredible boredom." She was soon discharged, and her mother came to stay with her to help as she slowly recovered.

Emily has a rocky relationship with her mother, mostly because they are in many ways exact opposites. Emily is rational and analytical, but her mother has a very different view of the world. She has at times worked as a spiritual counselor, and she believes nature can cure many ailments. She would do research on the internet and implore her daughter to try unusual treatments such as special diets or bee sting therapy. While bee sting therapy was once a fad treatment for MS, suggesting this to Emily makes little sense as she is allergic to bees. Nevertheless, her mother insisted that Emily would be cured if she could endure the massive welts.

These types of treatments are not uncommon in MS. By its very nature, MS is so variable and unpredictable that there are literally hundreds of purported cures. Personally, I believe the most worthwhile alternative treatment to pursue is dietary modification. Based on limited evidence, I recommend patients keep a whole-foods plant-based diet low in saturated fat and refined sodium. However, I must concede I have limited confidence in this approach. Every time I have an older patient who is doing well despite having had MS for several decades, I make it a point to ask about lifestyle habits, and ninety percent of these patients with relatively benign MS eat a standard American diet.

Emily would acquiesce to her mother at times and tried things such as the Terry Wahls' diet. However, she would lose patience after a while, and as a doctor and a patient, she is skeptical of unproven treatments. Her mother, on the other hand, objected to many standard medical therapies.

She thought steroids were bad for me. She thought plasmapheresis actually was okay except for having the catheter placed. I'm like, "What would you have me do?" I'm pretty sure she would have me lie in a bed and have someone pray or shake crystals over me.

Despite the disagreements, Emily was in good hands. Having assistance, company, and a loving family member were much appreciated. Her husband Michael also came to stay with her for a period. Michael's mother had multiple medical problems and died young, so Michael grew up seeing his father as the caretaker for his mother, and it was only natural for him to be the caretaker for his partner. But Emily and Michael would often clash as Emily insisted on being independent despite having obvious limitations.

He took a week of sick leave to come down, and he was really mad at me because I don't like asking for help. There's one time I was taking a nap, and I woke up feeling hungry and thirsty. So, I go to the kitchen to get a glass of water and a snack. Well, the doors were closed because we have these pocket doors. With my ataxia and what not, I couldn't get the door open and stay standing because I didn't have the coordination. He hears a thud. Of course, I mumbled to myself, and I'm cursing, "Why didn't you ask for help? Why are you such an idiot?" He comes, and he stands there in the corner, and he goes, "Really? I'm in the other room. I'm not sleeping. Can't ask for help?" I'm like, "Yeah, well…shit happens." That's who I am. I have bruises on my butt. It's okay.

Becoming disabled, even temporarily, has a way of providing a new perspective on life. At the time, Emily had an interest in pursuing a career as a neurocritical care specialist. Neurocritical care is an inpatient subspecialty that involves treating acutely and often severely ill patients with neurological diseases such as stroke, head trauma, and brain hemorrhage. It can be emotionally and physically taxing with high stress, long hours, and constant drama. For anyone, this career would entail tremendous lifestyle sacrifices, and with the specter of MS, Emily had to think very seriously. Unlike those confronting more predictable and controllable health conditions or traumatizing life events, people with MS often lack confidence in the future. Most of us experience what psychologists refer to as "safety signals" or learned cues that guarantee the absence of an aversive event[5]. With MS, there are no such guarantees.

> During that admission, I had conversations with myself and my family. "Can I do neurocritical care if I end up in a wheelchair?" Yes, I will improve, but someday, I may not. This is the first time I had to deal with that. So, based on that, I remember saying, "I can't be in a wheelchair and be intubating someone." Because of that, I decided to not do neurocritical care...based on that fact alone.

She was still quite impaired when she left the hospital, and she was off work for six weeks, missing about fourteen overnight calls which she later had to make up. Working one hundred hours a week is the punishment for getting sick or pregnant when you are a medical resident. This is why I took zero sick days over four years of residency. None of the other residents were eager to pick up the slack—when people are struggling themselves, they are not in the mood for charity—so she ended up brokering her own absence and arranging the schedule. Only one of the other residents never gave her any resistance, and she returned the favor by taking an extra call for him later on.

Emily was stuck at home for a while, but she gradually improved to where a casual observer would not notice the slightest hint of disability. She was lucky to bounce back because not everyone does, but to this day, she still has some residual symptoms. She has urinary urgency, the feeling that you need to get to the bathroom very quickly when you feel the urge. Fatigue plagues her at times, though not necessarily more than the typical doctor. Her left leg and foot are a bit weak and clumsy, and she will notice that her left shoe is disproportionately worn because she will catch her foot on stairs or other obstacles. If she walks on a treadmill, she feels a lack of fluidity in the left leg after a while. Here is a screen shot from one of Emily's MRI scans:

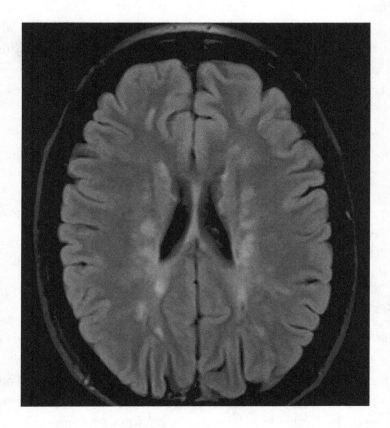

Figure 1: a T2 axial FLAIR image of an MRI scan of Dr. Emily Spitz in 2016 revealing multiple demyelinating lesions typical of multiple sclerosis.

Despite her relapse, she continued to endure the long hours and harsh lifestyle of a medical resident. She has a stellar reputation as a physician, and she sacrificed her elective time to complete her residency on schedule despite the prolonged absence. She diverted from the neurocritical care path and instead pursued additional training in stroke and vascular neurology. This is another subspecialty known for its masochistic lifestyle and cowboy mentality. Dr. Lyons actually advised she consider a career with a slower pace and daytime hours in case she were to worsen later in life, but Emily has a natural attraction to stroke and hospital-based care. She also figures if she becomes more physically disabled, she can always limit her hours or work from home as there are opportunities to care for stroke patients remotely in the rapidly evolving field of "telestroke."

There's a whole telestroke system in place in case I need it. I also really enjoy stroke, so this just dovetails into it. I would like to eventually be the director of a hospital program or an integral part of the administrative staff. I like knowing how a system works and trying to find ways to make systems better. I like teaching, so if I could get into a system where I'm in residency education, I would love that. That being said, I would like to have the ability to transition into a position that works for me if I'm not able to do a full sixty hour a week gig.

I have confidence I will find something that works for me. I also have the idea in the back of my head that I need to make sure I have a nice nest egg set aside in case I'm not able to work. The bigger concern—this is the one I don't think about—is what if I have cognitive issues so I can't actually do my job? That's like the worst-case scenario: what if I can't think? What if my knowledge evaporates? I just recently got disability insurance which is a little more expensive than what would be available for someone who doesn't have a condition, so that's the "in case things happen" plan.

I'm trying to prepare my life so I can continue to do my life. I want to be able to work as long as I can. Why? Because I put all this time, training, and effort into learning how to do what I'm doing. If I'm in a wheel-

chair, I can still do my future job. Will that be unfortunate? Yes. Will I deal with it? Yes. Because what are your other options? I don't consider myself an optimist. I think you have to deal with the hand you're dealt.

I think part of why Emily succeeds is her ability to downplay her condition and her symptoms. She thinks of herself as "normal," and she avoids blaming non-specific symptoms on MS. One problem with having MS is every bout of fatigue or cognitive shortfall gets attributed to the condition. In reality, we can consider some minor symptoms such as these universal vicissitudes of life. When you are fatigued, is this because of poor sleep, poor diet, stress, lack of exercise, random fluctuation, or the lesions in your brain? We never know which view is correct, but we always know which view is useful. Optimism is more valuable than realism sometimes. As is common with MS, Emily experiences significant day-to-day variation in her symptoms. Sometimes, she is more fatigued, less focused, or has mild weakness in the left leg. She disregards these small changes.

Residents are in many ways at the bottom of the food chain. Secretarial work, administrative arbitrage, and other undesirable tasks fall on you heavily. "Shit rolls downhill" is the adage. Despite all this, Emily is not the type to complain. When her service is busy, she grits her teeth and picks up the pace. If she has to stay up into the early hours of the morning to see a hospital transfer, she takes care of it as she would for any other patient. When she is working, she appears neither joyful nor miserable—just neutral and content. She has a hard-nosed sense of duty. It is not that she is emotionless. She feels depressed at times and wonders why she is so unlucky when she has a string of busy call nights. However, she tries to control her reaction to these emotions. She focuses on the task at hand and sets small short-term goals. She expects to have difficulties along the way and thinks experiencing struggle and making sacrifices is part of the natural course of being a doctor.

When I let myself focus on the negative side of life, I feel worse overall. That's a well-known phenomenon. If you feel bad for yourself, your muscles are sore. Everything feels crappy. I'm always looking ahead, and I think that allows me to bounce better. If I have something happening next week I have to get prepared for, it allows me to ignore the little details on the side I don't need to focus on.

In a way, having a neurological condition can be an advantage. Emily does not take her health for granted, and she has much deeper insight than the typical neurologist into what it subjectively feels like to have a neurological disease. She knows what it is like to be afraid and dependent on other people. Her experience makes her more empathetic and influences her approach to patients. Part of the reason she is such a perfectionist is that she has herself been seriously ill and has placed her trust in medical professionals to do everything right. At other times, she tells me that her MS ironically makes her less empathetic. Sometimes, she becomes frustrated when patients have minor or benign complaints.

Even though Emily's diagnosis is not a secret, she would not typically disclose she has MS to her patients. However, when she forms a particularly close relationship or thinks a patient would benefit from hearing about her experience, Emily feels comfortable sharing her story. She once had a twenty-one-year-old girl whom she diagnosed with MS. Even though the girl was doing well physically, the emotional impact of the diagnosis crushed her. She felt her life as a "normal person" was over and thought she would never have a romantic relationship, succeed in her career, or have children. Her mother would usually be present during the visits, but on the third or fourth visit, the patient's mother was parking the car, and Emily took the opportunity to talk to her about her own experience. It relieved the patient to see someone who had MS for over ten years who was so calm, successful, and formidable. It helped her to accept and come to terms with the diagnosis, and it inspired her to think more optimistically.

Emily has undoubtedly touched many lives during her tenure as a neurology resident, but she is moving to another state to obtain further training in the field of stroke at a new institution. She will continue to be in a long-distance relationship with her husband, a seemingly never-ending saga. I understand the sacrifice in doing this as I was in a cross-country relationship with my wife for two years when she left for graduate school. Emily would like to settle down and have children someday, but her career ambitions force her to go where her opportunities take her. Sadly, this is a common scenario for doctors, especially those in small subspecialty fields.

As I got to know Emily over time, I became increasingly impressed with her achievements and her attitude towards work. I wondered to myself, "How is she able to do it? What makes her unique?" She does not consider herself particularly optimistic, and she does not do anything specifically to improve her psyche. She exercises and does yoga for stress relief once in a while. However, she lacks the time to pursue hobbies or to seek out talk therapy for her depression. She is not religious, and she does not have much in the way of family or friends around her locally. Her coping skills seem to come naturally, and in her view, there is simply no other way. She does credit her parents for encouraging her and teaching her to work hard, and she especially recognizes her father as a role model for perseverance in the face of adversity.

In this book, I will interview four other people with MS, and we will look into some underlying mechanisms that may engineer one's response to conflict in life. Is this something which is intrinsic to the personality and cannot be manipulated? Is this the result of early childhood experiences or parental influences? Is this something we can manufacture, change, and enhance? Must one simply be tough like Emily, or are there other factors at bay? Even before I started researching or writing this book, I suspected the answers may be very complex and unique to each individual. In the next chapter, we will examine the abundant scientific research on the subject of resilience.

CHAPTER 2 REFERENCES

1. Vermersch P. Interferon beta-1a (Avonex TM): clinical and MRI impacts. Rev Neurol (Paris). 1999;155 Suppl 2:S13-9.
2. Lublin FD, Cofield SS, Cutter GR, Conwit R, Narayana PA, Nelson F, Salter AR, Gustafson T, Wolinsky JS, CombiRx Investigators. Randomized study combining interferon and glatiramer acetate in multiple sclerosis. Ann Neurol. 2013 Mar;73(3):327-40.
3. Jayne O'Donnell. Drug makers use co-pay coupons to help mask rising drug prices. USA Today May 3, 2017.
4. Rachel Z Arndt. High U.S. drug prices cannot be explained by R&D spending alone. Modern Healthcare March 7, 2017.
5. Christianson JP, Fernando ABP, Kazama AM, Jovanovic T, Ostroff LE, Sangha S. Inhibition of Fear by Learned Safety Signals: minisymposium review. J Neurosci Oct 10 2012; 32 (41): 14118-14124.

CHAPTER 3:
THE SCIENCE OF
RESILIENCE

"Indeed, this life is a test. It is a test of many things—
of our convictions and priorities, our faith and our faithfulness, our
patience and our resilience, and in the end, our ultimate desires"
—Sheri L Dew, *Saying It Like It Is*

RESILIENCE IS THE general ability to survive hardship and succeed in the face of adversity. Because of the significance and ubiquitous nature of this subject, plentiful amateur and scientific literature has been written about it. Whether or not you have MS, you will face difficulties in life which will test your resilience. You may become ill, lose a loved one, have turmoil in your career, or face any number of other challenges. This is the nature of modern life. However, many people, including those I interviewed for this book, do incredibly well despite significant adversity. Resilience is a generalizable skill that goes far beyond MS, and the good news is that we can improve and train it. It takes time to develop, and resilient people do not simply manage to avoid failure; rather, they turn failure and strife into something good. Resilience is a complicated trait with many components because real life calls for different skills and attributes in different situations. In the book, *The Resilience Factor* by Karen Reivich and Andrew Shatte, the authors state that resilience contains seven separate factors[1]:

1. Emotion regulation
2. Impulse control
3. Realistic optimism
4. Causal analysis
5. Empathy
6. Self-efficacy
7. Reaching out.

These factors provide a useful framework for discussing resilience, and we will refer to them throughout this book and see how they apply to my patients. We will review each of these concepts in some detail and learn how they contribute to resilience in the sections below. As I said, these attributes can be developed and nurtured, so they should not be thought of as intrinsic or unchange-

able. For developing resilience, Reivich and Shatte suggest strategies such as introspection, putting adversity into perspective, and
managing one's emotional response to remain calm and focused.
Keep in mind that few people are strong in all seven areas[1, page 2].

EMOTION REGULATION

Emotion regulation is taking control of your internal feelings. It is
one of the foundational components, because if you cannot control
your emotional response to the external environment, being resilient is nearly impossible. It is important to curb the natural tendency to worry excessively and ruminate in response to negative life
events. You should temper negative emotions like guilt, envy, and
anger. At the same time, you can accentuate and call to use positive emotional responses such as pride, hope, empathy, gratitude,
and humor. This ability develops early in childhood[2] and evolves
throughout life.

> *"As I walked out the door toward the gate that would lead to my free-
> dom, I knew if I didn't leave my bitterness and hatred behind, I'd still
> be in prison."*—Nelson Mandela

IMPULSE CONTROL

Closely related to emotion regulation is impulse control. Impulse
control is the capacity to suppress inappropriate behavioral responses. We all have compulsions to take actions which would sabotage
our relationships and long-term goals. We all know people who
have quit a job, moved to a new city, entered a romantic relationship, or started a new venture on impulse. This kind of behavior has
its advantages in helping people to break out of inactivity, but im-

petuous spontaneity is counter to the slow adaptations necessary for true resilience. Adjusting to major life events is gradual and requires deep-seated changes in outlook, abilities, and behavior patterns. In many situations, the right decision may be unnatural and counter-intuitive, so we should think before we act.

In the famous Stanford marshmallow experiment in the 1960s, psychologist Walter Mischel studied the phenomenon of impulse control and delayed gratification in young children. Researchers left children aged three to five in a room with a single marshmallow and told them they would receive two marshmallows if they waited fifteen minutes without eating the single marshmallow. The children who controlled their impulse to eat the sugary treat later had less behavior problems[3]. They were viewed as more competent as adolescents[5] and scored higher on the SAT by two hundred and ten points[3,4]. Those who ate the marshmallow immediately, however, had more difficulty handling stress and maintaining friendships. As adults, they had a higher body mass index and reported more problems with drugs[3].

"The ability to subordinate an impulse to a value is the essence of the proactive person." —Stephen Covey (The 7 Habits of Highly Effective People)

REALISTIC OPTIMISM

Even in the face of difficult times, it is important to forge a realistic optimism. This is the process of maintaining a good outlook in the context of what we can reasonably expect. It is not only the optimism to imagine a better future but also a way of looking at your current situation to bring positive things to light. If you believe the future will be better, you are more likely to make decisions that will make this a self-fulfilling prophecy. If this is your worldview, you are more likely to work harder, maintain a better diet, exercise regularly, and interact with people more enthusiastically. Optimistic people have more willpower[6] for this reason. The positive emotions generated by optimism reduce stress and allow you to broaden your focus and put things into perspective[7]. However, this optimism about the future must be reasonable, or else reality will dash your expectations and crush your psyche. After a hard day at work, did you have two rude customers or forty-eight friendly customers? Did the restaurant have poor service or was the meatloaf excellent? Is the rain annoying or refreshing? It is all in your head. As a neurologist, I mean this literally: your perception of the world is a manifestation of the mushy, gelatinous structure in your cranial vault, not the external environment.

"A pessimist sees the difficulty in every opportunity; an optimist sees the opportunity in every difficulty" — *Winston Churchill*

CAUSAL ANALYSIS

The next concept of resilience is that of causal analysis, the logical process of determining the cause of the adversity. Not all problems in life can be solved by positive thinking, gushy proverbs, and a supportive therapist. Sometimes, we must take a step-by-step analytical approach and figure out where we are going wrong. When I was a third-year medical student, my rotation in internal medicine quickly turned into a miserable grind. I would stay up late studying, sleep four hours, and sluggishly toil through the day—stressed, fatigued, and in poor spirits. After a few weeks, I reflected and judged sleep was more valuable than knowledge in my performance on the wards. I set a simple bedtime, and the difference was night and day. I was instantly more energetic and focused, and this proved more valuable than book knowledge in the hospital. The solution will not always be so straight forward, but you may find it if you look hard enough for it.

"By three methods we may learn wisdom: First, by reflection, which is noblest; second, by imitation, which is easiest; and third by experience, which is the bitterest." —*Confucius*

EMPATHY

Empathy is feeling the emotions that others feel. Although empathy would seem a trait more geared towards helping others, it is actually crucial in forging one's own resilience. The reason for this is surviving the hardships of life highly depends on developing supportive relationships. This in turn requires an understanding of other people's feelings, emotions, and experiences. There is also an ineluctable connection between empathy and having insight into our own emotions[8, page 96]. Empathetic people have richer and more meaningful friendships; they have closer bonds with family members. Empathetic people find it easier to seek support and to reach out.

"Empathy is about standing in someone else's shoes, feeling with his or her heart, seeing with his or her eyes. Not only is empathy hard to outsource and automate, but it makes the world a better place." — *Daniel H. Pink*

SELF-EFFICACY

The idea of self-efficacy is the endpoint of multiple other foundational principles as it is the confidence to survive misfortune and to enact change in your life. It is having faith in one's own ability to face challenges and solve problems. Self-efficacy relates to the psychological principle of the locus of control. Some people view themselves as acting on the world, and others view the world as acting on them. This dichotomy represents the internal versus the external locus of control. Depressed people use a paradigm with an external locus of control[9] which is dangerous because it is inherently pessimistic and promotes idleness. To have self-efficacy is to believe you have both the opportunity and ability to accomplish a task at hand. This belief itself is powerful. It was Henry Ford who said, "Whether you think you can or you can't, you're probably right."

To some extent, our attitude towards self-efficacy and the locus of control may have to do with our life experiences. In early experiments on learned helplessness, American psychologist Martin Seligman studied two groups of dogs[10]. One group was exposed to random electric shocks which they could not escape. Another group of dogs was exposed to electric shocks which could be stopped by pressing a lever, and the dogs in this group quickly learned how to press the lever in response to a shock. Then, both groups of dogs were placed into a new scenario where the dogs could escape the electric shock by jumping from one part of the apparatus to another. The dogs who had been exposed to the lever were much more likely to learn the new adaptation. The dogs who were taught "learned helplessness" simply stayed idle and whimpered when they were shocked. This same theory applies to humans[11]. If you are exposed to experiences early in life in which you cannot escape negative consequences, you might be less likely to have self-efficacy. If this is true, I implore you to gain insight and to fight against this tendency.

"It always seems impossible until it's done." — *Nelson Mandela*

REACHING OUT

The last principle of resilience is reaching out which is putting yourself out there to exploit the positives in life and to pursue new ventures. In the famous self-help book, *The 7 Habits of Highly Effective People*, Stephen Covey argues interdependence, not mere independence, produces the highest level of productivity. Almost all the great achievements in human history are related to cooperation between groups of people. I could not practice medicine in its current form without physicians in other specialties, nurses, phlebotomists, radiology technicians, and medical assistants. Less directly, I depend on computer scientists, electrical engineers, construction workers, and individuals with various other skill sets. Nobel Prizes are often split between multiple researchers in different disciplines. Human resources are the greatest asset of any corporation. We must have the ability to not only take advantage of our own strengths but also the collaborative strengths of everyone around us. We must be willing to try new things and to develop novel ambitions, challenging ourselves and fearlessly risking failure.

"No man is an island, entire to itself; every man is a piece of the continent" — *John Donne*

Naturally, people are stronger in some components of resilience and weaker in others. Even in areas where people appear to be strong, they may falter at times. If I am to look at someone like Dr. Emily Spitz from the previous chapter, she has many of these features, but she is far from perfect. She is generally in control of her emotions and is certainly not impulsive. However, she does suffer from depression and became noticeably distraught during her major relapse. She shows us resilience is not the same as stoicism or emotional immunity. She does not describe herself as being optimistic, but she is practical and realistic. At the very least, she is optimistic about herself and her future, at least in so far as she knows she will adapt to whatever challenges she faces. She has self-efficacy and causal analysis in abundance. Her empathy has served her well in strengthening her relationships with other people. Despite all her problems and fears, she has reached out to the point of pursuing her career, making new friends, and trying new things.

When I was interviewing Emily, I assumed her resilience came from her hard-working parents and her upbringing. However, Reivich and Shatte argue that early childhood experiences and genetics are not as important as we presume[1, page 11]. To be sure, some factors correlating with resilience are beyond our control. Risk factors for lower resilience include low birth weight, poverty, low parental education, a troubled family structure, and abuse[1, page 16]. However, these things in addition to our education and opportunities may be less important than certain aspects of our cognitive style. We form this cognitive style over decades, and it can be quite malleable. Some people, for instance, have a systematically pessimistic style of thinking. Other people jump to conclusions or are quick to blame others for their problems[1, page 13]. Sometimes, we may erroneously believe a specific problem is a general character fault[1, page 108]. If Emily believed that she would not persevere, would she do all the little things necessary to stay afloat? If she assumed she would not recover from her major relapse, would she be as aggressive in seeking treatment? If she blamed her colleagues for not being more accommodating, would she be willing to work as hard? We must analyze and eliminate counterproductive thoughts if we are to be resilient.

ICEBERGS

Some people have deep-seated and often unconscious beliefs which can hamper their progress. Reivich and Shatte call these beliefs "icebergs" because they may appear small but are massive below the surface. For instance, Emily treated the twenty-one-year-old patient I described in the last chapter who believed a diagnosis of MS meant the definitive end to all her dreams. This was, in effect, an iceberg, and when Emily broke apart this belief by telling her own story, everything became much easier. Icebergs tend to relate to perceptions of achievement, social acceptance, and independence[1,

^{page 125-127}. For instance, Emily believes asking others for help is a sign of weakness, and she believes strongly in independence and self-reliance. This iceberg is harmless most of the time, but it caused significant trouble during her major relapse, and it could be problematic if she were to become disabled later in life. She is still in the process of addressing this iceberg.

People with MS commonly have hidden icebergs which result from societal stereotypes about the illness. I had a patient in her early thirties tell me she never dated because she thought no one could love someone with MS. I told her that most of my patients are in happy relationships with supportive partners. Many young people with MS with significant and visibly apparent disability get married and have children. I had a high school student who was devastated because he thought MS meant the end of his football dreams. I encouraged him to continue his training, and he went on to play for a prominent college team. I have had countless patients ask me if they should give up on a particular career path because of the diagnosis. Surely, these are reasonable and practical thoughts to have, but they can be more harmful than good. Unless my patient wishes the impossible, my advice is always the same: pursue your dreams. Everyone has thoughts like these, so it is very important to be introspective. What is your cognitive style? What are your icebergs? Are these thoughts justified and helpful or unreasonable and counterproductive?

ME VS. NOT ME, ALWAYS VS NOT ALWAYS, AND EVERYTHING VS. NOT EVERYTHING

Another aspect of cognitive style is the way we interpret negative events in our lives. We can blame events on ourselves, or we can blame them on other people or our circumstances. We can view these events as unique instances or as recurring problems. We can see conflict as affecting only a single aspect of life or as being pervasive and universal. Reivich and Shatte call these ways of thinking "me vs. not me," "always vs not always," and "everything vs. not everything"[1, page 153]. For instance, I recently had a case where I had overlooked a key finding on an MRI scan. Was this because of my error, or was the radiologic finding very subtle? Was this a rare event, or am I incompetent at reading MRI scans? Does this problem relate only to interpreting a specific MRI finding, or am I deficient as a clinician? Every situation is unique, but people tend to be biased towards a certain subconscious explanatory style. If you are a "me, always, everything" type of person, you blame everything on yourself and view deficiencies as chronic and broad. With this mentality, you are likely to view minor misfortunes as catastrophic. If you are a "not me, not always, not everything" type of person, you are likely to trivialize your mistakes, defer blame, and fail to learn from misjudgments. It is important to be accurate and flexible in your interpretation of events so you can respond appropriately. Excessive optimism can be just as harmful as pessimism which is why optimism must be qualified with realism.

The key to building resilience, according to Reivich and Shatte, is to be introspective and to develop a resilient cognitive style over time. You also must learn to control your emotions and to manage stress with other techniques such as controlled breathing, progressive muscle relaxation, positive imagery, and meditation[1, page 192-198]. Use causal analysis to approach problems logically and flexibly, and you will build confidence and self-efficacy. You can then reach out and pursue new ambitions without fear and self-doubt. Reivich and Shatte have designed resilience training programs to help children, those with psychological problems, salespeople, and corporate managers. Resilience is also important for romantic relationships and for parenting. Rigorous scientific studies support their methods and show a correlation between resilience and real-life outcomes. They also demonstrate the ability to improve resilience with specific training.

MEASURING RESILIENCE

Resilience is very difficult to measure. It has been described in many ways in different contexts by different people. It is not a singular phenomenon but rather an amalgam of related traits like self-reliance, meaning, equanimity, and existential tranquility[12]. Research studies generally use brief questionnaires, and there are at least fifteen separate metrics ranging from the dispositional resilience scale (1989) to the Child and Youth Resilience Measure (CYRM, 2008)[13]. No single gold-standard measure of resilience exists, and the items in the scales are highly subjective and perhaps mood-dependent. However, they are often subjected to validation studies.

In 2015, Rüya-Daniela Kocalevent and colleagues published a population-based study on resilience using face-to-face surveys of 5,036 Germans[14]. The metric used was the RS-11, an eleven-item questionnaire each with a seven-point Likert scale. Just to give you a sense, these are the items on the scale (rated 1-7 from "No, I disagree" to "I agree completely.")[15]

1. When I make plans, I follow through with them
2. I usually manage one way or another
3. Keeping interested in things is important to me
4. I feel that I can handle many things at one time
5. I am friends with myself
6. I am determined
7. I keep an interest in things
8. I can usually find something to laugh about
9. I can look at a situation in a number of ways
10. Sometimes, I make myself do things whether I want to or not
11. I have enough energy to do what I want to do

Many of these statements mirror the concepts of resilience described by Reivich and Shatte. Items #1 and # 10 relate to impulse control; #3 and # 7 relate to causal analysis; #5 relates to emotion regulation; #8 relates to realistic optimism; #9 relates to reaching out; finally, #2, #4, #6, and #11 relate to self-efficacy. They report that resiliency is positively associated with self-esteem (R=0.66) and with life satisfaction (R= 0.47) but is inversely associated with depression (R = -0.4) and anxiety (R= -0.32). Men and women had roughly equal average resiliency scores, and there were no clear differences based on age, marital status, level of education, employment, or household income.

I gave the RS-11 survey to everyone I interviewed, and the full results are listed in **appendix C**. To be honest, I always find these surveys to be a little silly because it is too obvious what the "correct" answer is (that is, the answer that signifies resilience). I tried to minimize bias by having them fill out the surveys prior to the interview and by giving no prompt except to say, "Please fill this out as honestly as possible." Here is how Dr. Emily Spitz (Chapter Two) responded to the RS-11 (her selections in bold):

1) When I make plans, I follow through with them
   I strongly disagree I disagree I disagree somewhat undecided/neutral I agree somewhat **I agree** I agree strongly
2) I usually manage one way or another
   I strongly disagree I disagree I disagree somewhat undecided/neutral I agree somewhat I agree **I agree strongly**
3) Keeping interested in things is important to me
   I strongly disagree I disagree I disagree somewhat undecided/neutral I agree somewhat **I agree** I agree strongly
4) I feel that I can handle many things at one time
   I strongly disagree I disagree I disagree somewhat undecided/neutral I agree somewhat **I agree** I agree strongly
5) I am friends with myself

I strongly disagree I disagree I disagree somewhat undecided/neutral I agree somewhat **I agree** I agree strongly

6) I am determined
   I strongly disagree I disagree I disagree somewhat undecided/neutral I agree somewhat I agree **I agree strongly**

7) I keep an interest in things
   I strongly disagree I disagree I disagree somewhat undecided/neutral I agree somewhat **I agree** I agree strongly

8) I can usually find something to laugh about
   I strongly disagree I disagree I disagree somewhat undecided/neutral I agree somewhat **I agree** I agree strongly

9) I can look at a situation in a number of ways
   I strongly disagree I disagree I disagree somewhat undecided/neutral I agree somewhat **I agree** I agree strongly

10) Sometimes, I make myself do things whether I want to or not
    I strongly disagree I disagree I disagree somewhat undecided/neutral I agree somewhat **I agree** I agree strongly

11) I have enough energy to do what I want to do
    I strongly disagree I disagree I disagree somewhat undecided/neutral I agree somewhat **I agree** I agree strongly

---

POST-TRAUMATIC STRESS DISORDER

The concept of resilience has been specifically studied in various contexts. For instance, South Korean men entering obligatory military service are required to take the Korea Military Personality Test (KMPT). This test is given at about age nineteen and assesses various psychological metrics including the seven resilience factors described by Reivich and Shatte. It also evaluates early life stress defined by physical, emotional, or sexual abuse, neglect, or exposure to domestic violence. As expected, early life stress was associated with depression, anxiety, and aggression—a pattern seen in other studies[16]. However, higher resilience scores were found to mitigate the effect of early life stress on creating these psychopathologies. Out of the seven characteristics, emotion regulation had the largest effect of minimizing the negative influence of early life stress.

A large body of evidence suggests your personality and life experiences prior to a major life event will affect your resilience. In 2011, Erika Wolf published a study on eighty-six war veterans with post-traumatic stress disorder (PTSD) and its association with personality traits[17]. The severity of PTSD was associated with having a generally negative temperament ($r=0.54$) as measured by personality scales. PTSD has been associated with alcohol and drug use as well as underlying psychiatric conditions such as depression, schizophrenia, and personality disorders[18]. Indeed, about half of PTSD sufferers have concomitant major depression[19]. Part of this may be due to shared risk factors as both PTSD and depression are linked to childhood adversity and abuse[20]. Previous trauma or assault, particularly at a young age, is another risk factor for developing PTSD[21]. In a meta-analysis of multiple studies on the risk of veterans developing PTSD after combat done by Chen Xue et al., the following were found to be associated with a higher risk of PTSD[22]:

1. female gender (OR 1.63)
2. ethnic minority status (1.18)
3. low education (1.33)
4. non-officer rank (2.18)
5. Army service (2.3)
6. combat specialization (1.69)
7. two or more deployments (1.24)
8. longer cumulative length of deployments (1.28)
9. prior adverse life events (1.99)
10. prior trauma exposure (1.13)

11. prior psychological problems (1.49)

12. trauma severity (2.91)

13. deployment–related stressor (2.69)

14. discharging a weapon (4.32)

The number in parentheses above (x.xx) is the odds ratio which is the increased risk relative to those without that risk factor. For instance, those who discharged a weapon in service had a 4.32-fold higher risk of PTSD compared to those who had not. Some of these factors relate to the stressor itself such as #5–#8 and #12–14. Several factors such as age, marital status, and socioeconomic status had no clear effect. Support for the victim's unit and post deployment support decreased the risk of PTSD. Some studies have found younger soldiers are at increased risk of developing PTSD[23].

Personal factors related to resilience have a tremendous effect on the risk and prognosis of PTSD as well. In studies of trauma victims, about ten percent of trauma survivors develop PTSD[24]. However, those with an optimistic outlook fare better than those with a more pessimistic outlook. Furthermore, people with an active rather than passive coping style have better recovery from PTSD. Active coping involves facing problems and emotions head on rather than viewing yourself as a passive victim. This is analogous to the internal versus external locus of control which we discussed in relation to the idea of self-efficacy. In addition, people who are flexible in their thinking do better than those who are cognitively rigid.

CHILDHOOD

Part of resilience in response to trauma may relate to early childhood experiences. Those subjected to severe and overwhelming stressors are more susceptible to PTSD. However, people with a history of overcoming mild and manageable stressors such as family relocation, romantic breakups, or unemployment may be more resistant to PTSD[25]. Perhaps the major traumas induce a sort of learned helplessness found in Martin Seligman's dogs exposed to inescapable shocks. In contradistinction, comparatively minor and controllable early traumas are analogous to a vaccination which induces immunity to future, more significant traumas. Manageable adversity teaches us to experience new emotions and to learn new skills. If we look at the history of Dr. Emily Spitz, we can see she did have some early "microtraumas." Her father had a disability, and her family overcame financial difficulties. Emily also had to confront her own mother after an affair. These experiences may have served as "practice exacerbations," preparing her for future clinical exacerbations from MS. She was also lucky she recovered quickly from relapses early in her illness, giving her a sense of optimism. She may have fared much worse if she had developed a major attack like the relapse she suffered during her residency while she was still a teenager.

These early life experiences undoubtedly influence resilience, but they do not appear to be the final word. Many people arise from extraordinarily unfavorable circumstances and go on to demonstrate remarkable strength of character. The American developmental psychologist Emmy Werner and her colleague Ruth Smith conducted a forty-year study on 698 infants born in 1955 on the Hawaiian Island of Kauai[26]. About a third of the infants had significant risk factors for a poor developmental outcome such as poverty, mental illness in the family, or an unstable household. Many of these disadvantaged children grew up around violence, alcoholism, and other forms of strife. Often, they went on to have problems of their own such as criminal behavior, teenage pregnancy, and poor mental health. However, about a third of these children became highly competent, well-adjusted, and resilient adults despite their backgrounds. What the children with more favorable outcomes had in common was they were more likely to have a strong relationship with someone outside the nuclear family such as a distant relative or a teacher. They were also more likely to participate in a religious or community group. This demonstrates that resilience is a complex and evolving trait with multiple contributors.

Even if your background is more favorable than these children of Kauai, our modern hyper-connected society will always provide us with ample sources of stress and turmoil. This is easy to see in the local environment, but even problems in the greater society can affect our emotions and test our resilience. After the terrorist attacks on the United States on September 11, 2001, there was a wide-spread increase in psychological disturbances. This was true even for people who live far from New York and knew no one directly affected by the attacks[27]. I was a college freshman at UC Berkeley at the time, and I remember the disturbed look on people's faces and the unusually quiet campus. Nationwide, many people reported crying spells[28], depressive symptoms, trouble sleeping, and cognitive problems[29].

Despite all these negative emotions, the 9-11 attacks provided an opportunity for resilient people to turn the tragedy into something positive. Because there was a shared national grief, many people felt more connected to their family members and their community. Most Americans reported strengthening of personal relationships after the attacks[30]. Interest in politics and international affairs increased, and many popular songs had a nationalistic and hopeful message. What is it that allowed people to survive and thrive in the face of fear and uncertainty? According to University of Michigan psychologist Barbara Fredrickson, resilient people can generate positive emotions in the face of adversity to promote preservation of psychological resources and personal growth[27].

BROADEN AND BUILD

In a study done by Fredrickson on University of Michigan students and alumni before and after the September 11th attacks, forty-seven participants underwent detailed psychological testing to evaluate the effect of resilience, personality, and other factors on psychological outcomes. Students commonly expressed fear, anger, disgust, difficulty studying, and anxiety, but these reactions were unassociated with resilience scales done prior to the attacks. However, resilience correlated with optimism and tranquility after the attacks. The ability to find a positive meaning from the aftermath and to generate pleasant emotions correlated with a good psychological outcome. Many students later reported feelings of gratitude, love, and pride. The more resilient students were less neurotic, less depressed, and reported greater overall life satisfaction. These data show us that resilience is not an immunity to troublesome life events; it is the capacity to find a silver lining in a cloud of calamity.

The ability to turn a tragedy into something positive is not a rare phenomenon. Many American prisoners during the Vietnam War reported the experience enhanced their appreciation for life and strengthened their connections with family members[31, page 10]. People can often take a step back to look at the big picture, broadening their perspective, refining their values, and changing their path in life. Frederickson calls this the "broaden and build" theory of positive emotions[31, page 34].

Resilience has also been studied in various other populations and situations. It is important after a divorce for both the parents and children[32]. After a natural disaster, the resilience of individuals has a tremendous effect on the recovery of the community[33]. There is also an element of group resilience whereby cooperation, communication, and altruism can be more important than individual grit. This has been researched extensively in survivors of hurricane Katrina in the Mississippi Gulf Coast[34-36]. Resilience also has a critical influence on coming to terms with the death of a loved one and allowing family members a healthy bereavement and an ability to move on with life[37].

BIOLOGICAL FACTORS

Unsurprisingly, resilience has some identifiable biological markers. One study measured the blood levels of neuropeptide-Y and de-hydroepiandrosterone (DHEA) of U.S. Army soldiers undergoing special training for high-pressure interrogations. These substances limit the release of hormones such as cortisol and norepinephrine in response to stress, blunting the "fight or flight" response. The trained soldiers had higher levels of DHEA and neuropeptide Y immediately after an interrogation compared to soldiers who had not undergone the training[38]. Other forms of evidence corroborate the importance of these hormones. Animal studies have shown that injecting neuropeptide-Y directly into the amygdala ameliorates anxiety and promotes resistance to stress[39]. Carriers of a gene which leads to lower neuropeptide Y production experience greater anxiety and amygdala activation in response to a threatening stimulus[40].

The downstream mediators of the stress response such as norepinephrine are important as well. In an experiment by Larry Cahill and James McGaugh at the University of California, Irvine, subjects were shown a series of pictures and given either placebo or propranolol, a drug used to treat high blood pressure which blocks the effects of norepinephrine in the cardiovascular system and other tissues. Subjects in the experiment receiving propranolol were less likely to remember pictures showing disturbing images compared to controls receiving placebo, purportedly due to dampened emotional activation[31, page 47]. The same effect was demonstrated by testing the memory of emotionally arousing stories[41]. Oxytocin, the hormone associated with love, social behavior, and childbirth seems to have a similar effect of attenuating the hypothalamic-pituitary axis and promoting resistance to chronic stress[42]. A natural stress response is adaptive and important for survival, but an overwhelming response is harmful. Every individual is different, and our response to stress seems to result from a complex interaction between our genes and environmental factors[31, page 18].

I cannot overstate the harmful effects of chronic stress on the body. Chronic stress can cause various physical symptoms such as diarrhea, weight gain, suppression of the immune system, elevated blood pressure, and poor cognitive function[43]. According to research by Dr. Amy Arnsten at the Yale neuroscience lab, chronic stress can impair working memory and executive function. High levels of norepinephrine released during chronic stress may alter the physiology in the prefrontal cortex by binding low-affinity α_1 and β_1 norepinephrine receptors[44]. The prefrontal cortex is important in complex planning and decision making, and its finely tuned function allows us to define goals, anticipate problems, and navigate social situations. As opposed to low levels of norepinephrine seen in normal alertness, high norepinephrine impairs neuronal firing and leads to lower working memory performance[45, 46].

The following figure shows the stress response and some biological factors related to it:

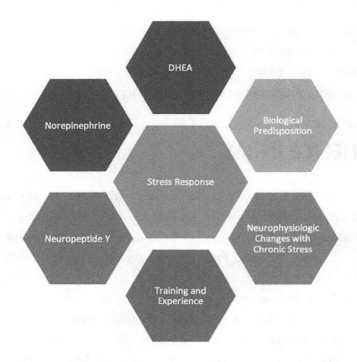

Figure 1: The Stress Response

People with MS can find themselves in a cycle of chronic stress, fear, and negative consequences. If chronic stress is causing physical ailments and poor cognitive function, it is difficult to make progress. Part of being resilient is learning to break the cycle and to mitigate the harms of chronic stress. Just because the stress response is biological does not mean it is unmodifiable. Research shows us that the brain is much more plastic than we imagined. After years of practice, a violinist can increase the surface area of the motor cortex used to control her playing hand. Expert divers develop specific anatomical adaptations as well. They have increased cortical thickness of the right parahippocampal gyrus, the right orbitofrontal cortex, and the left superior temporal sulcus[47]. These regions relate to memory, sensory processing, and decision making[48-50]. It is not such a giant leap to believe we can modify the anatomy and physiology of our brains to make ourselves more resilient. Emily Spitz demonstrated some features of resilience right from the start of her MS diagnosis, but you will see from the other stories that resilience often develops more gradually over many hard-fought years.

RESILIENCE IN MS

Scientific studies on resilience in people with MS have shown us how to tailor the principles of resilience to the specific hardships of the disease. In 2015, Black, et al. published an online survey of 196 people with MS and found a positive affect and self-efficacy were the strongest predictors of resilience in MS[51]. The symptoms of MS will naturally sabotage self-confidence and provide plenty of reasons for negativity, so it is important to counteract this.

In a Northeastern metropolitan MS clinic, a nonrandomized trial was conducted on thirty-five people with MS in which the subjects would receive multidisciplinary treatments designed to improve resilience. They received services such as social work, counseling, and nursing[52]. They also received physical and occupational therapy. The intervention addressed not just psychological factors such as depression and coping but also pragmatic limitations like fatigue, mobility, and social isolation. Instead of following a regimen, they tailored the therapies to individual needs. They gave the patients resilience surveys before and after the eight-week intervention, and there was an improvement from an average raw score of 123.8 to 139.6 on the RS14 resilience scale (p < .001). A control group of nine patients had no change in resilience. On the pre-treatment test, higher income was linked to greater resilience, but in the post-treatment test, the income gap disappeared. The authors note that loneliness and social isolation are prevalent in the MS community[53], and we know that social support relates strongly to resilience and self-perceived health status[54, 55]. An impressive element of this study is the comprehensive nature of the intervention. It is not enough to simply try to feel better despite having MS; one has to learn to work through and live with limitations in the real world. The very act of doing this is empowering.

I do not intend to suggest that you can achieve everything with ease if you are resilient enough. The purpose of this book is not to imply that we can overcome any physical suffering with some sort of Zen-like mysticism. Disease, disability, resilience, and social institutions interact intricately, and each person's experience in the world is unique. We are all entangled in a web of complicated traits and relationships, and what works for one person will not work for another. Some influences of outcomes in people with MS are shown in the bubble chart below:

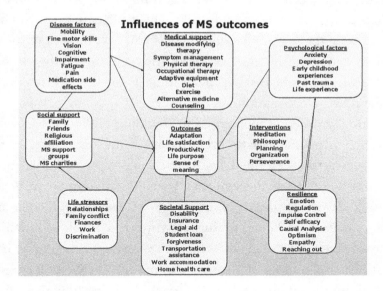

Figure 2: Influences of psychological outcomes in multiple sclerosis

Although it would be ideal for everyone with MS to receive continuous assistance and support from a highly trained multidisciplinary group, this is rarely practical in the real world. Because of this, many proponents of the field of positive psychology have attempted to create self-directed and small group programs to bolster resilience. For instance, Dr. Dawn Ehde and Dr. Kevin Alschuler from the University of Washington have developed a positive psychology program called "everyday matters"[56] for people with MS[A] They believe it is a misconception that success is the main determinant of happiness, and they claim that happiness is a choice which we can develop and foster with specific goal-directed behavior. They encourage meditation and journaling along with altruism and the regular expression of gratitude. Strengthen relationships with old friends, join networking groups, pursue hobbies, or take part in charity events. Do not underestimate the importance of an active and fulfilling social life. Long-term and imposing goals should be broken down into smaller and easily achievable components. They also propose the "twenty second rule." If you have an idea of something you want to do, start acting on this within twenty seconds, even if the action is as trivial as writing it down and arranging a separate time to pursue the idea further.

Naturally, different techniques for building resilience will work for different people. Nearly everyone has some weaknesses in the resilience factors described by Reivich and Shatte. Think about where you are strong and where you would like to improve. When facing a setback in health or in life, try to use the "broaden and build" paradigm and focus on turning your troubles into something positive. Recognize that while happiness and resilience are partly situational and biological, they are also modifiable. We will explore more about the different schools of psychology and how they apply to individual resilience in Chapter Five. In the next chapter, we will hear the incredible and inspiring story of Dr. James Bhat.

A   For more information about the program, go to https://www.nationalmssociety.org/Resources-Support/Library-Education-Programs/Everyday-Matters.

CHAPTER THREE REFERENCES

1. Reivich K, Shatte A. The resilience factor: Seven essential skills for overcoming life's inevitable obstacles. New York: Broadway Books, 2002.
2. Harris, P. L. Children's understanding of the link between situation and emotion. Journal of Experimental Child Psychology, 1983;33:1–20.
3. Lehrer, J. Don't; The secret of self-control. The New Yorker. May 18 2009:6-32
4. Mischel W; Shoda Y, Rodriguez, MI. Delay of gratification in children. Science 1989;244.
5. Shoda Y, Mischel W, Peake, Philip K. Predicting Adolescent Cognitive and Self-Regulatory Competencies from Preschool Delay of Gratification: Identifying Diagnostic Conditions. Developmental Psychology 1990;26(6):978-986.
6. Bernecker, K Job, V. Beliefs about willpower moderate the effect of previous day demands on next day's expectations and effective goal striving. Front Psychol 2015; 6:1496.
7. Fredrickson BL. The role of positive emotions in positive psychology. The broaden-and-build theory of positive emotions. Am Psychol;2001;56(3):218-26.
8. Coleman, D. Emotional Intelligence. Bantam, 2006.
9. Benassi V. A.; Sweeney, P. D.; Dufour, C. L. Is there a relation between locus of control orientation and depression? Journal of Abnormal Psychology 1998;97(3): 357–367.
10. Seligman M. E. P. Learned helplessness. Annual Review of Medicine 1972;23(1): 407–412.
11. Rigoli F, Pezzulo G, Dolan RJ. Prospective and Pavlovian mechanisms in aversive behaviour. Cognition 2015 Nov 2;146:415-425.

12. Wagnild G; Worden, MT. The Resilience Scale: Users Guide for the US English Version of the Resilience Scale and the 14-Item Resilience Scale (RS-14). The Resilience Center, 2009.

13. Windle G, Bennett, KM, Noyes, J. A methodological review of resilience measurement scales. Health and Quality of Life Outcomes 2011;9:8.

14. Kocalevent RD, Zenger M, Heinen I, Dwinger S, Decker O, Brähler E. Resilience in the General Population: Standardization of the Resilience Scale (RS-11). PLoS One. 2015 Nov 2;10(11).

15. von Eisenhart Rothe A, Zenger M, Lacruz ME, Emeny R, Baumert J, Haefner S, Ladwig K. Validation and development of a shorter version of the resilience scale RS-11: results from the population-based KORA–age study. BMC Psychology 2013, 1:25.

16. Scott KM, McLaughlin KA, Smith DA, Ellis PM. Childhood maltreatment and DSM-IV adult mental disorders: comparison of prospective and retrospective findings. Br J Psychiatry 2012;200:469–475.

17. Wolf EJ, Harrington KM, Miller MW. Psychometric properties of the Schedule for Nonadaptive and Adaptive Personality in a PTSD sample. Psychol Assess 2011 Dec;23(4):911–24.

18. Wolf EJ, Harrington KM, Miller MV. Psychometric Properties of the Schedule for Nonadaptive and Adaptive Personality in a PTSD Sample. Psychol Assess 2011 Dec; 23(4): 911–924.

19. Flory JD, Yehuda R. Comorbidity between post-traumatic stress disorder and major depressive disorder: alternative explanations and treatment considerations. Dialogues Clin Neurosci. 2015 Jun;17(2):141-50.

20. Gilbert R, Widom CS, Browne K, Fergusson D, Webb E, Janson S. Burden and consequences of child maltreatment in high-income countries. Lancet 2009 Jan 3; 373(9657):68–81.

21. Breslau N, Chilcoat HD, Kessler RC, Davis GC. Previous exposure to trauma and PTSD effects of subsequent trauma: Results from the Detroit Area Survey of Trauma. American Journal of Psychiatry 1999;156:902–907.

22. Xue C, Ge Y, Tang B, Liu Y, Kang P, Wang M, Zhang L. A Meta-Analysis of Risk Factors for Combat-Related PTSD among Military Personnel and Veterans. PLoS One 2015;10(3):e0120270.

23. Booth-Kewley S, Larson GE, Highfill-McRoy RM, Garland CF, Gaskin TA. Correlates of posttraumatic stress disorder symptoms in Marines back from war. J Trauma Stress 2010 Feb; 23(1):69–77.

24. Haglund M, Cooper N, Southwick S, Charney D. 6 keys to resilience for PTSD and everyday stress. Current Psychiatry 2007 April;6(4):23–30.

25. Khoshaba DM, Maddi SR. Early experiences in hardiness development. Consulting Psychology Journal: Practice and Research 1999;51(2):106–16.

26. Werner E. E. Vulnerable but invincible: a longitudinal study of resilient children and youth. New York: McGraw-Hill, 1989.

27. Fredrickson BL, Tugade MM, Waugh CE, Larkin GR. A prospective study of resilience and emotions following the terrorist attacks on the United States on September 11th, 2002. Journal of Personality and Social Psychology 2003;84 (2): 365–376.

28. Saad, L. Personal impact on Americans' lives: Women express much more fear of terrorism than do men. Gallup news service 2001.

29. Swanbrow D. Institute for Social Research How America responds: Part 2. University of Michigan News Information Service, 2001.

30. Saad L. Americans anxious, but holding their heads high: Have increased confidence in government leaders, the economy. Gallup news service, 2001.

31. Southwick S, Charney D. Resilience: The science of mastering life's greatest challenges. Cambridge University Press, 2012.

32. Hopf S.M. Risk and Resilience in Children Coping with Parental Divorce. Dartmouth Undergraduate Journal of Science 2010.

33. Heyzer N. Building Resilience to Natural Disasters and Major Economic Crises. UN ESCAP, 2013.

34. Lee J, Blackmon BJ, Cochran DM, Kar B, Rehner TA, Gunnell MS. Community Resilience, Psychological Resilience, and Depressive Symptoms: An Examination of the Mississippi Gulf Coast 10 Years After Hurricane Katrina and 5 Years After the Deepwater Horizon Oil Spill. Disaster Med Public Health Prep 2017 Aug 30:1-8.

35. Blackmon BJ, Lee J, Cochran DM Jr, Kar B, Rehner TA, Baker AM Jr. Adapting to Life after Hurricane Katrina and the Deepwater Horizon Oil Spill: An Examination of Psychological Resilience and Depression on the Mississippi Gulf Coast. Soc Work Public Health 2017 Jan 2;32(1):65-76

36. "The emotional cost of distance: Geographic social network dispersion and post-traumatic stress among survivors of Hurricane Katrina"; Morris KA, Deterding NM; Soc Sci Med. 2016 Sep;165:56-65.

37. Greeff AP.; Human B. Resilience in families in which a parent has died. The American Journal of Family Therapy 2004;32: 27–42.

38. Morgan CA, Wang S, Southwick SM, Rasmusson A, Hazlett G, Hauger RL, Charney DS. Plasma neuropeptide-Y concentrations in humans exposed to military survival training. Biol Psychiatry 2000;47(10):902-9.

39. Jeilig M, Koob GF, Ekman R, Britton KT. Corticotropin-releasing factor and neuropeptide Y: role in emotional integration. Trends Neurosci 1994;17(2):80-5.

40. Zhou Z, Zhu G et al. Genetic variation in human NPY expression affects stress response and emotion. Nature 2008 Apr 24;452(7190):997-1001.

41. Cahill L, Prins B, Weber M, McGaugh JL. Beta-adrenergic activation and memory for emotional events. Nature 1994 Oct 20;371(6499):702-4.

42. Stanić D, Plećaš-Solarović B, Mirković D, Jovanović P, Dronjak S, Marković B, Đorđević T, Ignjatović S, Pešić V. Oxytocin in corticosterone-induced chronic stress model: Focus on adrenal gland function. Psychoneuroendocrinology 2017 Jun;80:137-146; 2017 Mar 10.

43. McEwen B, Sapolsky R. Stress and Your Health. J Clin Endocrinol Metab 2006;91 (2): E2.

44. Arnsten AFT. Stress signaling pathways that impair prefrontal cortex structure and function. Nat Rev Neurosci 2009 Jun; 10(6): 410–422.

45. Birnbaum SB, et al. Protein kinase C overactivity impairs prefrontal cortical regulation of working memory";; Science. 2004;306:882–884.

46. Arnsten AFT, Mathew R, Ubriani R, Taylor JR, Li B-M. α-1 noradrenergic receptor stimulation impairs prefrontal cortical cognitive function. Biol. Psychiatry 1999;45:26–31.

47. Wei G, Zhang Y, Jiang T, Luo J. Increased Cortical Thickness in Sports Experts: A Comparison of Diving Players with the Controls. Plos One 2011 Feb 16;6(2):e17112.

48. Ferreira NF, de Oliveira V, Amaral L, Mendonça R, Lima SS. Analysis of parahippocampal gyrus in 115 patients with hippocampal sclerosis. Arq Neuropsiquiatr 2003 Sep;61(3B):707-11.

49. Kringelbach M. L. The orbitofrontal cortex: linking reward to hedonic experience. Nature Reviews Neuroscience 2005;6: 691–702.

50. Senkowski D, Schneider TR, Foxe JJ, Engel AK. Crossmodal binding through neural coherence: implications for multi-sensory processing. Trends Neurosci 2008 Aug;31(8):401-9.

51. Black R, Dorstyn D. A biopsychosocial model of resilience for multiple sclerosis. J Health Psychol 2015 Nov; 20(11):1434-44.

52. Falk-Kessler J, Kalina JT, Miller P. Influence of Occupational Therapy on Resilience in Individuals with Multiple Sclerosis. Int J MS Care 2012 Fall;14(3): 160–168.

53. Beal CC, Stuifbergen A. Loneliness in women with multiple sclerosis. Rehabil Nurs 2007 Jul-Aug; 32(4):165-71.

54. Bonanno GA, Mancini AD. The human capacity to thrive in the face of potential trauma. Pediatrics. 2008 Feb; 121(2):369-75.

55. Krokavcova M, van Dijk JP, Nagyova I, Rosenberger J, Gavelova M, Middel B, Gdovinova Z, Groothoff JW. Social support as a predictor of perceived health status in patients with multiple sclerosis. Patient Educ Couns 2008 Oct; 73(1):159-65.

56. Everyday Matters; Living Your Best Life with MS; Using the Principle of Positive Psychology to Manage the Challenges of Living with a Chronic Illness. available at http://www.nationalmssociety.org/NationalMSSociety/media/MSNationalFiles/Documents/Everyday_Matters_SHG_Participant_Workbook_Final.pdf

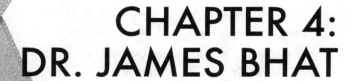

CHAPTER 4:
DR. JAMES BHAT

"The greatest glory in living lies not in never
falling, but in rising every time we fall."
— Nelson Mandela

I ORIGINALLY MET JAMES Bhat when one of my colleagues referred him for a second opinion. He has had MS since 2006 and has unfortunately developed a very significant degree of physical disability over the last twelve years. He walks slowly and awkwardly with a walker but requires a wheelchair for long distances. The instability of his torso and his wide stance remind one of a toddler first learning to walk. Thankfully, he is lean and fit, else gravity might make walking impossible. He has "scanning speech," a soft and uncoordinated voice which is a sequela of cerebellar dysfunction. His handwriting is illegible on bad days, and he experiences double vision at times. His disability is instantly recognizable to everyone he meets, and a layperson could easily mistake him for having cognitive impairment because of his slowed and unusual speech. Everything he does takes longer and is more labored.

When we first met, I reviewed his extensive history, and we discussed new and unexplored options. I was also naturally curious about his background and lifestyle. He is calm, friendly, and easy to talk to—the quintessential type B personality. A stereotypical "armchair professor," James likes to ponder about a subject slowly and deeply. He is the opposite of Emily Spitz in many ways. I imagine that he would have the same countenance if he were completely healthy or bed-bound. What I found fascinating about James is that he seems to be impossibly high functioning. He works part time as a psychiatrist. He has a wife and two sons. He comes to his appointments alone and manages his life, his practice, and his medical care without much assistance. I thought to myself, "How could he still be working?", and I wondered about the logistics. He approaches MS very differently from Emily, and he changes the way we think about disability and resilience. This is the story of James, his history of MS, and how he continues to struggle and thrive.

James was born in Las Vegas, Nevada. His parents came from a traditional Indian background, but his childhood was far from conventional. His parents divorced when he was four, and he lived with his mother until about age ten. They later moved to Dallas to live with his new step-father. At age fourteen, he left to live with his biological father in New York where he went to high school.

It was kind of a tumultuous thing where I was being shuttled around—family to family—never really that comfortable because it was always changing. It wasn't really something I could feel too comfortable with. I always felt like the third wheel.

James has two half-brothers eight and ten years younger than him, and he has a step brother ten years older than him. He has no full siblings, and he has never lived with relatives close to him in age. It was also hard for him to maintain long term childhood friendships because of his family situation, so he spent very little time with friends until he was in high school in New York. He had a good relationship with his parents and his stepfather, but it was not without complications.

My mom, in general, is just very quiet and passive. That's just her deal. She was a very loving mom and would always do what I needed from her and that kind of thing. My dad passed away about five years ago. He was an alcoholic, and so for him, he was totally fine when he was sober, but when he was drinking, you never knew what he was going to be like. He could be really angry. He could be really jovial. It was just…you didn't know. I still remember, he would get very angry at me, and it was totally nonsensical. I was like, "Why?" He had a lot going on in his life.

After his parents divorced, James's father remarried and lived in Las Vegas for a long time. He then divorced again and married a third time, but his relationship with his third wife was rocky, and he was alone much of the time. As James describes it, his father's isolation was significant enough to be a factor in his tragic death. He died after a head injury that occurred when he was drunk and had an accidental fall. He was alone at the time and was only discovered later on. James was thirty-two at the time.

James's stepfather had a military background and was very strict. The entire family valued academic achievement, so James found that focusing on his studies was a natural and practical way to stay out of trouble and pass under the radar. His parents were not excessively harsh or punitive, but a pristine report card has a way of silencing naggers. He was intelligent and diligent, performing well from as early as the sixth grade. Academics came easily to him. He was not the type to become apprehensive or fretful; he just did the work. It was part of his "MO" as he puts it. In his family's culture, profession and institutional history define a large part of one's value and character. His father specifically encouraged him to go into medicine from a very young age.

His whole thing was, "You're going to be a doctor. You're going to be a doctor. You're going to be a neurosurgeon." I don't even think he knew what that was.

We shared a laugh when he said that. People sometimes think doctors choose specialties to fatten their wallets and impress people at parties. I cannot imagine that this would make up for spending forty years working without passion. You would have to drag me kicking and screaming into a neurosurgery residency program. James commiserated with me that he never understood this aspect of Indian culture. That people should have concrete goals independent of their individual personality and tendencies is unreasonable to him, and he does not bestow this value onto his children. James has no doctors in his immediate family, but medicine was respected and encouraged nonetheless. He initially went along with it and fortunately ended up liking it.

I firmly believe that once you do medicine, there's enough stuff in medicine that you can choose something that really suits you. So for me, I like psychiatry, right. If psychiatry wasn't in the cards, then yeah—maybe I wouldn't like medicine, you know.

His studious habits led to a circle of friends full of like-minded individuals. He lived in an urban area but attended a private high school full of ethnic well-heeled future engineers, computer scientists, and doctors. It was, without a doubt, a haven for nerds and geeks. He has always had a certain attraction to people who are in some way disenfranchised—people who seem to get the short end of the stick. He identifies with them. However, he never truly felt at home in Long Island, and when he packed up his car to leave, he took every single thing he owned, leaving absolutely nothing behind. He was trying to start anew and find his own way.

James ended up pursuing an abbreviated combined undergraduate and medical school program through Stony Brook University School of Medicine (SUNY). SUNY allowed a student to complete undergraduate and medical school in only six years. Entrants would finish their undergraduate requirements in only two years, and they would automatically be funneled into the Stony Brook University School of Medicine provided they maintain certain grades and other metrics. These programs are notoriously competitive to enter, and they attract a specific type of student: someone who has seemingly planned their whole life or has had their whole life planned for them by their parents (see **appendix A** for an example).

I used to interview such applicants at my alma mater, Drexel University College of Medicine. They looked like little kids to me and appeared uncomfortable and awkward in their silly suits. I admired their ambition, but it was hard to take them seriously as medical school applicants. I was immature enough at age twenty-one when I started medical school. I cannot imagine starting at nineteen. SUNY has since changed their program to a seven-year program, perhaps learning that life experience is as important as book smarts.

In the Indian mindset, the faster the better. So, that place—because it was six years—was full of Indian people, and so that was my cohort. I ended up just having a bunch of friends that were Indian. Because it was a six-year thing, you didn't really have a choice—you just studied and fulfilled the requirements. There was a little bit of humanities and stuff like that, but it was mostly science. I ended up with a BS in biology. Not to sound cocky or whatever, but all that stuff wasn't very taxing for me...I mean I could do it. So, I did it, and it never caused me too much sweat.

It is natural to feel a kinship with those who have the same background, challenges, and ambitions, so James formed a social group primarily with people in the SUNY program and later with those in his medical school class. He studied hard, but he had some time for a social life. Through hobbies such as basketball, painting, and other creative activities, he made ample friends, and he reflects on this time with nostalgia. Nothing was too dramatic or eventful; it was par for the course.

Perhaps because of the urgings of his father, James initially was interested in pursuing a career in surgery. He became close friends with a Bangladeshi cardiothoracic surgeon who had moved to the US to pursue research in the field. James ended up taking part in this research, and he at one point was seriously considering a career in cardiothoracic surgery. It was not until the third year of medical school during his clinical rotations when he discovered an interest in psychiatry.

He was drawn more to the therapy aspect of psychiatry rather than the pharmacologic aspect. The Northeast has a reputation of a fast paced and less humanistic style of medicine, but James feels that the exact opposite is true in psychiatry. His mentors in New York were not simply cerebral physiologists and prescription scribblers, and this influenced his approach to the field. Prescribing medications for psychiatric conditions can become somewhat robotic. For depression, there are antidepressants. For bipolar disorder, there are mood stabilizers. For schizophrenia, there are antipsychotics. Take into account clinical characteristics, medical comorbidities, dose, route, compliance, and side effects. Rinse and repeat. It is complicated but ultimately a one-size-fits-all approach. You do not prescribe Zoloft© instead of Prozac© based on your patient's early life experiences or current multifactorial stressors. Serotonin is the same molecule in everyone. James likes therapy because it is more thoughtful, intellectual, and nuanced.

The summer between his second and third year of medical school also encouraged James to pursue psychiatry. The good thing about being twenty-two and single is that you feel no pressure to take a linear path. He requested an academic leave and stayed with an old college friend in Seattle. Through bartending and other odd jobs, he saved up enough money for a plane ticket to India. He stayed there for several months and gained experience in Ayurveda, an alternative system of medicine popular in India[1]. Ayurveda literally means "life-knowledge," and the practice emphasizes balance and a holistic approach. He was not in a formal training program, but he worked with various Indian doctors in different regions. He saw a sampling of styles and flavors, and he also observed the practice of western medicine in India. To some extent, the principles of Ayurveda are reflected in his current practice. We can see this holistic style in a statement found on his commercial website:

In order to be truly happy, we must strive for balance. This is stressed in eastern philosophy but is often not a part of traditional western medicine. Without living a balanced life, it can be quite difficult to be fully happy and content. Dr. Bhat believes that psychotherapy can help us break patterns that repeatedly cause us to be unhappy and help us build new patterns that can help us reach a more balanced place. Often times, it is necessary to incorporate a number of different modalities to pave the way to reaching our goals without being impeded by our past.

James finished the last two years of medical school and joined a residency program in psychiatry at Los Angeles County Hospital affiliated with the University of Southern California Keck School of Medicine. I am familiar with the institution because I worked there as a research tech in an andrology lab between high school and college. It has a famous trauma center and a large underserved immigrant population. People like the program because you have the opportunity to help the truly needy, and you will be respected as a physician on your first day of internship. The pace is fast and unpredictable. Trauma, late presentations of chronic diseases, and unusual characters dominate the emergency room. The Internal Medicine residents have a post-it board boasting the most outrageous lab values of patients who survived to discharge. I remember seeing absurd numbers that seemed physiologically impossible or foreboding of certain death. The record for Hemoglobin was 1.8 g/dl which has a normal range between 12 and 17.5g/dl. This represents a ~85% loss of red blood cell mass which would be fatal in most circumstances.

Needless to say, the environment was perfect for someone looking to see interesting cases and to work with incredible people. James loved psychiatry, and he enjoyed both his residency program and his lifestyle in Los Angeles. He made several new friends and had enough time to socialize and reap the benefits of living in a thriving hip city. Many students from USC medical school would do rotations in psychiatry at LA Country Hospital, and among them was James's future wife.

I met James's wife briefly. She is now an oncologist, and we coincidentally have a loose connection in that she supervises the infusion center where some of my patients receive treatment. The world is amazingly small. Friendly, gregarious, and confident, her personality stands apart from James's quiet disposition. She has a certain formidability that reminds me of Emily Spitz. Given everything he has been through, James is lucky to have a strong woman in his life. I would guess she was the ruler of the household long before James became disabled. She has an ability to stay organized, to notice the little things, and to clean up loose ends. In describing their relationship and the differences between their personalities, he makes an analogy using a colander (a cooking pot).

So basically, my colander has really big holes, and her colander has really small holes. My nature is that a lot of things will pass through my colander. My holes are really big, so I don't have a lot of plans, but I'm fairly confident she does. My whole thing has been that I can always let everything pass through my colander because I'm confident that whatever I should care about is going to be caught in her colander.

There was a point in life where James seemed to be the luckiest guy in the world. He got engaged near the end of his residency to a beautiful woman with a shared culture and a mutual passion for medicine. All of his years of hard work and sacrifice would begin to pay off in increased autonomy and financial security. Medicine is the ultimate quest of delayed gratification. When you are so close to your goals, it is impossible not to be hopeful and optimistic in anticipation of the future. You think about maxing out your 401k, buying a house, and splurging on various luxuries. You think about practicing in your own unique style without meddlesome attendings. You think about forming lifelong relationships with patients. You think about beginning a research career, starting an entrepreneurial venture, or otherwise making a name for yourself.

I think the one thing I always remember is that I was at a friend's house, and we were playing volleyball. I went to jump and hit the ball, and I fell down. That totally took me by surprise because I'm a fairly decent athlete, and that was something weird. Why would that happen, you know? That was it; I fell. Nothing else really bothered me. The only other thing is that at that time, I had been going to yoga, and I noticed when I was doing some of the poses, my balance was off. It just seemed a little bit weird that I couldn't do some of those poses. It wasn't totally out of the norm. It was like, "This seems kind of weird."

The symptoms were extraordinarily subtle. He was neither numb nor weak. He could still do everything he wanted to do, but he noticed a slight imbalance and lack of coordination. More out of curiosity than concern, he ended up seeing a neurologist and having an MRI scan. Somehow, he ended up receiving a report of the MRI from the office staff, and he read it on his own without a physician present to offer explanation or consolation. This is definitely not standard protocol. Imagine believing yourself to have an innocuous symptom only to open your MRI report to find this doozy:

Numerous abnormal T2 hyperintense lesions are present in the brainstem, cerebellar peduncles, bilateral periventricular/subcortical region, and bilateral thalami without appreciable associated enhancement, compatible with history of demyelination. Ill-defined T2 hyperintensity in the posterior C1-C2 spinal cord is also noted on image 13 of series 4 without enhancement. Corpus callosal involvement is noted with thinning. There is questionable punctate/linear enhancement along the corpus callosum, best seen on image 12/22 of series 11 and coronal image 12/27 of series 12; vascular enhancement may contribute to the appearance also. Prominent ventricle and sulci. Minimal deviation of septum pellucidum to the left. Mild opacities in the visualized paranasal sinuses.

In other words, his MRI scan showed extensive abnormalities typical of MS in the brain and spine. They also found slight shrinkage of the brain. His films are shown below in Figures 1 and 2:

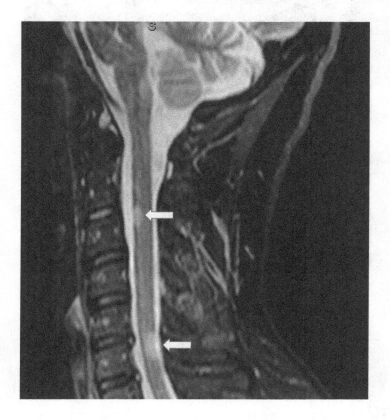

Figure 1: A T2 sagittal MRI of the cervical spine revealing MS plaques in the spine and medulla. A few of the lesions are denoted by arrows

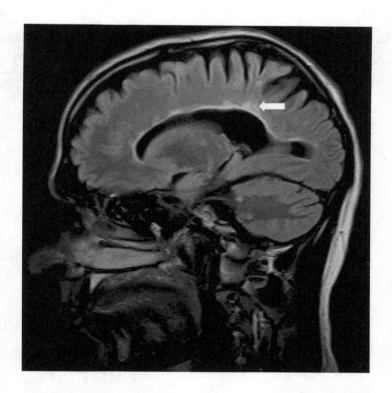

Figure 2: A parasagittal T2 FLAIR MRI of the brain showing MS plaques in the corpus callosum, subcortical white matter, and cerebellum. Some lesions are denoted by the white arrow.

I assure you being a doctor does not make this an easier pill to swallow. If anything, we are anxious patients with type "A" personalities. As they say, a little knowledge is a dangerous thing, and sometimes the imagination of a well-informed patient can run wild. I was nervous enough when my daughter had benign neonatal jaundice. As doctors, we have seen the worst of the worst, and we know the limits of allopathic medicine. However, James was more accepting than most, and he moved on with his life despite the shocking news and horrible timing.

That totally rocked my world for a good day or two. Over time, I guess I somehow tried to get around that whole thing. Looking back, I think what happened to me and probably happens to a lot of people is that there's just this sort of denial you have. Alright, I get it. I have MS or whatever, but I can do most of the things I could do otherwise. You really don't cognize it so much. Having been through that, I probably would have embraced that time—that good year or two or three—to do things I cannot do now.

James is not the sort of person to dwell on the past or worry about minute details, but he was active in pursuing the best medical care. He sought out a well-known MS specialist in the area, a respected academic known for writing books, publishing research articles, and speaking at conferences. He has trouble remembering all the details of his early MS history, partly because of his forward-looking outlook and partly because his early history was a whirlwind of relapses and medications.

Many times, MS can be surprisingly benign. Based on one cohort study, the median time from diagnosis to requiring a cane to walk one hundred meters was 27.9 years[2]. In other words, if we diagnose you at thirty, you have a fifty-fifty shot of walking independently at age fifty-eight. In the same study, only twenty-one percent required a cane fifteen years after diagnosis. To make things better, these patients were diagnosed prior to the development of any FDA approved drugs, and many of the newer disease modifying therapies are highly effective in relapsing MS. Unfortunately, James had very aggressive disease and did much worse than the average patient despite various treatments.

He was first treated with Betaseron© but had multiple relapses requiring intravenous steroids. His attacks came with worsening balance, clumsiness, double vision, and weakness. Follow up MRI scans showed an increased burden of lesions, and he switched to Copaxone©, but this failed to halt the relentless exacerbations and new MRI lesions. He received multiple courses of steroids, most providing incomplete recovery, and the attacks left him with worse and worse neurological function. Rebif© and Avonex© yielded equally poor results. He tried Ampyra© (dalfampridine), a medication used to improve walking function in MS, but it proved useless. All the injectable disease modifying therapies have comparable and modest efficacy, and they are often ineffective in aggressive relapsing MS. Because of this, people make treatment decisions based on convenience, insurance, and side effects.

The one thing my wife and I remember is that Dr. Ryu would always compare medications saying, "Six of one; half a dozen of the other," kind of like "it doesn't matter." So, there's six of one and half a dozen of the other. So, they're both the same. That would always get under my skin. That doesn't help me. I get it. I get it. What would YOU do in my situation?

His neurologist offered more aggressive options such as Cytoxan©, Novantrone©, and Tysabri©, and he did try a few rounds of Cytoxan© despite fearing the risks. But by 2009, three years after diagnosis, James was already walking with a walker. Think about this in the context of the fifty percent of patients who should be walking independently after twenty-eight years without the benefit of medical science. In modern times, it is less common to hear stories like this because there has been a trend in the field of MS towards earlier and more aggressive treatment. Vignettes like these make the risk of more potent drugs seem trivial, so doctors and patients are more willing to treat aggressively upfront.

In some sense, James was in denial about his worsening condition. He is not the type to think pessimistically, but this has both advantages and disadvantages. It makes it easier to focus on the vicissitudes of life and to make it through the day. On the other hand, it can predispose one to complacency and malaise. People often have a false sense of confidence in pharmaceuticals and medical doctors. I have seen patients demonstrate incredible loyalty to a drug despite the fact that they have objectively and dramatically worsened while taking it. Sometimes, it is important to be realistic about your situation and to be your own advocate.

It's hard to think about it because there's a part of you—I should say a part of me—that tried to think about things in a certain way in the moment to get by...in order to make things a little more palatable. But that may not be a very objective way of looking at things. You're asking me to be a little bit objective which totally makes sense, but that's kind of in contrast to the way I had to think in order to get by.

James did get by and continues to get by with amazing grace, but it was difficult to deny the gravity of his condition, so he began to take it more seriously. His wife was very involved in his care at this point. She would come to his appointments, ask many questions, and make suggestions. James would often "button up" during appointments and allow her to take the lead, and she advocated vigorously for him. When standard treatments are failing so indubitably, it is natural to look for alternatives, so they read the medical literature avidly and explored new options. After losing confidence in the traditional approach, they ended up pursuing a risky but promising alternative: hematopoietic stem cell transplant.

Stem cell therapy has a certain aura and mysticism around it. As I type the words "stem cell," you imagine undifferentiated cells forming new neurons and glia, sprouting dendrites, remyelinating damaged axons, and miraculously restoring lost function. Unfortunately, at the time of this writing, there is to my knowledge no good evidence demonstrating that stem cell treatments can regenerate lost neural tissue in MS. Nonetheless, hematopoietic stem cell transplant is unquestionably a well-established effective treatment of relapsing MS. In fact, we have had it for over forty years[3]. It just works differently than most people imagine. The way stem cell transplant works in MS is as follows:

1. Bone marrow is harvested from the patient
2. Toxic chemotherapy drugs are given to destroy the patient's native immune system
3. The bone marrow is replaced to restore and "reboot" the immune system.

There are many protocols, and some "stem cell" treatments do not require bone marrow transplant, but the concept is always the same. The theory is that you destroy the abnormal immune system and restart it, hoping that the new immune system lacks the prior inclination to attack the nervous system[4]. The chemotherapy drugs also provide a potent short-term immunosuppression which often improves recent inflammatory injury. Perhaps "immune system destruction therapy" would be a more accurate name than "stem cell therapy." However, you need not hire a marketing consultant to figure out which title would be more attractive to prospective patients.

After hematopoietic stem cell transplant, patients who have recently had a series of relapses will often improve, sometimes dramatically. Also, recipients will commonly enter long term remission, and they may remain stable for many years or even indefinitely without any additional therapies. In one case series published in JAMA[5], forty-one out of one hundred and forty-five patients receiving hematopoietic stem cell transplant for relapsing remitting MS had significantly improved at two years after treatment. Furthermore, 80% of patients had no relapses whatsoever during the four-year period after treatment. Sometimes, remission will be persistent, and other times, MS will appear to return after several years, but when it does, it may respond to more conservative treatments. The same effect of profound improvement or prolonged remission can occur if a patient receives chemotherapy for an unrelated cancer[6]. I have had a few young patients enter long term remission after receiving treatment for breast cancer.

Unfortunately, bone marrow transplant has never become a standard treatment of relapsing MS because of the unfavorable side effect profile. Harvesting bone marrow requires an invasive procedure. The chemotherapy drugs ablate the immune system, exposing the recipient to opportunistic infections. There are also the traditional chemotherapy side effects such as anemia, nausea, hair loss, and diarrhea along with a myriad of other possible consequences[5, 7, 8, 9]. Still, James was desperate, and his wife urged him to seek treatment with Dr. Richard Burt, a well-known hematologist at Northwestern University famous for the treatment of autoimmune diseases with bone marrow transplant. Dr. Burt is a controversial figure, but he seems to exercise reasonable restraint. He turns down patients who are poor candidates, and he is reluctant to use the word "cure."

They accepted James for the treatment in August 2009, and he flew to Chicago to stay with relatives. He received cyclophosphamide and anti-thymocyte globulin, two nasty chemotherapy drugs. This was followed by an inpatient bone marrow transplant, several supportive treatments, and a month-long hospitalization. The secondary effects were dreadful. He had the expected hair loss and nausea, but more significantly, he was weak and lethargic for several months. He took a huge step back and was severely deconditioned. His energy and focus were so poor he has no memory of many of the harrowing details. However, he improved somewhat over several months, and for a time, he could walk independently without a cane, though he still had significant limitations.

James went through extensive rehab, and he had to redo all his childhood and adult vaccinations because chemotherapy destroys memory lymphocytes. He was stable for a period, and he simply moved on with life. His work in private practice resumed, and he was eager to start a family. He had saved a semen sample prior to receiving chemotherapy because of the risk of infertility, but this proved unnecessary. He had his first son about a year after leaving Chicago. However, following a brief period of unadulterated optimism and no chronic pharmaceuticals, his relapses returned, and he again began to worsen. Retrospectively, he is not 100% confident the stem cell transplant provided him any benefit, and he was certainly worse off a few years after the treatment than he was beforehand. However, he feels that the severity of relapses and his rate of decline have attenuated in the last several years.

He changed health insurance shortly after coming back to Los Angeles and saw an Indian neurologist who is close friends with his wife's sister. They knew each other prior to their professional encounter as he had met her at kids' birthday parties and other family events. He was later seen by one of my colleagues and then by me in 2015. After Dr. Burt's treatment, he was doing well for a period and was not using any medication for about one year. After a relapse, he restarted the previously ineffectual Rebif© in 2010. He then changed back to Avonex©, another drug that had failed him in the past. In 2011, his speech worsened. In April 2012, he developed a flare with double vision and an eye movement disorder known as internuclear ophthalmoplegia. He received intravenous steroids but did not improve, and he was left with double vision when he looks to either side. In 2013, his wife gave birth to a second son. He has tried to live life as normally as possible, adjusting his daily routine along the way. His quest for a sustained remission continued, and he took Tysabri© (natalizumab) for a brief period. Then, he was on a combination of Avonex© and azathioprine, and most recently, he tried rituximab. During the last several years, he has also followed a Paleolithic diet. All in all, he is only modestly worse than a few years ago, and he is not the type to complain about subtle differences.

With all of the treatments, people ask me, "Do you feel this; do you feel that? Do you feel better?" I don't feel anything, and I will only tell you if I can dunk a basketball. That's how I will know that there is anything different. I'm very thankful in a way because a lot of what I want to do, I can still do. I can still be a psychiatrist.

James has been fortunate in a sense because he seems to be relatively unaffected by most of the common invisible symptoms of MS. His cognition is excellent, and he has been pain free most of the time. However, he does have a few MS-related problems which others cannot easily see. He has significant fatigue, and most things take him longer than they should, even accounting for physical limitations. During active tasks, his strength will often be adequate at first but then deteriorate quickly, forcing him to pace himself or look for alternate ways to accomplish simple chores. In 2016, he suffered a bout of trigeminal neuralgia, a recurrent excruciating pain in the face caused by dysfunction of the trigeminal nerve. People usually describe it as an "electric shock" rating "ten out of ten" on the pain scale, and eating, talking, shaving, or touching the face can trigger it. This condition is associated with MS, but it can also occur in isolation and often does not have an obvious cause. To treat the pain, James used seizure medications including Tegretol© (carbamazepine) and Trileptal© (oxcarbazepine) which ameliorated his symptoms but caused lethargy as a side effect. We fiddled and titrated the medications to a happy medium until the condition seemed to improve on its own.

It was a crazy terrible pain. It would last for a few seconds at a time, but if the pain is like a ten out of ten, a few seconds is still terrible.

Despite the trigeminal neuralgia, James did not have significant pain during most of his disease course. Much of his struggle is visibly clear to everyone he meets. This is an advantage in that no one could ever question the legitimacy of his disease. No one will ever think that he is imagining his symptoms, elaborating on their severity, or simply not trying hard enough. He has no significant brain fog, and he suffers from no psychiatric conditions. What you see is what you get.

James is the kind of person who is focused on the here and now. He does not fret over how things will be in five or ten years. I think this is helpful in his situation because the possibilities are endless, and the computations and uncertainties would be overwhelming. Still, I should not underestimate the day-to-day challenges James faces. He cannot drive, so he hires a driver to take him to and from work. He has a walker that can fold into a wheelchair, and on bad days, his driver will help him into his office. A baby monitor sits in his waiting room which lets him see and speak to patients from his office, calling them from afar instead of coming awkwardly to the door.

Even when sitting down with patients, the interaction is not entirely routine. He has an obvious speech disorder and speaks more slowly and laboriously than most. He has trouble writing prescriptions, and he will often have to call the pharmacy to explain his poor penmanship or simply call in the prescription. Occasionally, he will have to take a bathroom break during a session. He does not program extra time into his work day, and he rarely mentions his condition to his patients. Luckily, most of them treat him without prejudice so long as they are satisfied with the care provided, and his practice has been quite successful. This is all so incredible to me when I think about how many seemingly better-off individuals with MS cannot work due to factors such as pain, fatigue, frequent urination, or fluctuations of symptoms throughout the day. It is not uncommon for a thirty-year-old with MS with no major physical problems to be on disability based on a combination of invisible symptoms. James is truly exceptional in his ability to make the best of his situation.

I feel like I'm kind of on autopilot where I don't really think things could be so different. I just try to do what I do, and I don't think I'm making an active choice. I think it's always been a part of me to want to do what I can. If I didn't, it might be a very depressing place to be. I feel like throughout my whole life, I am dealt a hand of cards, and then I just make the most of what I have. God doesn't give you anything you can't deal with.

James's optimism and perseverance are especially impressive to me because I saw him as a patient and interviewed him during a particularly difficult time in his life. He and his wife have always been very different people, and a chasm has grown between them over the years. They simply have different approaches to interacting with the world. He is more introverted and takes the world as it comes. She is more sensitive to changes around her and more aggressive in her planning. Relatively speaking, he is "type B," and she is "type A." A lot of their early disagreements related to his medical care. In the beginning, she would go to all of his appointments and act as an assertive advocate. However, he took offense to this because he wanted to be autonomous and do things his own way. He became disenchanted with her domineering approach while she became frustrated by his nonchalance, and the clashes and stresses taxed both of them. They ultimately decided to let him manage his health care on his own, but he was resentful of the lack of support. It is difficult to look around a waiting room and realize you are one of the few people without an attendant.

It's always been a little bit weird just in that we're very different people. She, just by her very nature, is a concrete sort of person…which I can understand. You kind of have to be to some degree to have patients who are dying all the time, but that's just not my deal. I'm a psychiatrist.

I personally have fallen victim to his wife's mindset. It is very hard to be sensitive to the worldview and complaints of others when you deal with tangible and objective suffering. This experience changes your perspective irreversibly. This can be a good thing in that it makes you more grounded and appreciative of what you have, but it has negative consequences. I cannot react to stories of rude waitresses and missed bus rides in the same way. It is like giving a chocolate bar to a heroin addict; it is insufficient to cause arousal. This is why doctors sometimes appear cold, uncaring, arrogant, and heartless. We are overly practical and have a dark sense of humor. It is easier and less emotionally weighty to have some degree of detachment. I have to consciously remind myself that not everyone has the same standpoint.

MS can put a tremendous strain on romantic relationships. I have seen my patient's partners show admirable loyalty and make the most incredible sacrifices for their beloved. However, I have also seen arguments, breakups, and divorces. I remember one patient's spouse would castigate him by saying, "Are you going to use the MS excuse again?" Physical disability in general[10] and MS in particular[11] are known to increase the risk of divorce. This is logical because many causes of increased family stress including poverty[12], alcoholism[13], and religious differences[14] are linked with divorce. It has even been reported that participating in a clinical trial could increase the risk of divorce by focusing attention on the medical condition and exposing marital dissatisfaction[15]. Interestingly, there is some evidence that men are more likely to leave their wives than the other way around. One study found that a woman is six times more likely to be separated or divorced shortly after a diagnosis of cancer or multiple sclerosis than if the man had the condition[16]. Who knew we were so disloyal? Maintaining a happy marriage in which both partners feel mutually respected and cared for is difficult enough, so imagine adding the additional tension of a serious medical condition.

James and his wife have recently planned to separate, and as I write this, they are still working out the details. The decision was mutual, and there are no fixed long-term plans. He is thinking about moving into an apartment nearby, and family members will help him take care of his children. He and his wife interact pleasantly, and the arrangements are being made without malice. James views it as a new chapter in life, something he can manage just like any conflict he has ever faced. Still, he is understandably distraught.

When he told me about the impending separation, I could not help but balk because it was not what I expected. He is someone who seems to have everything together. When I entered his home, I found it beautiful and organized. He and his wife were friendly and cordial. His two children, now aged six and three, were joyful and energetic, running about the house looking for new adventures with youthful exuberance. I noticed they had an entire section of a massive living room filled with toys, and I commented, "It looks like they get everything." James agreed. His elder son said, "Not everything," but James rebutted by asking, "Tell me something you wanted that you didn't get?" They met this with wide-eyed silence. Everything about his home and his family felt perfectly harmonious, yet under the surface, it is so troubled. Even the most privileged and competent are not immune to marital difficulties.

Despite all the struggles with his health and in his personal life, James has been astonishingly resilient. He truly has all the features Karen Reivich and Andrew Shatte describe as components of resilience. He is emotionally stable and not impetuous. He is hopeful and confident yet pragmatic. He is logical and looks to understand his problems, yet he is empathetic to others. He is a very capable person, but he knows when to ask for help and how to exploit the surrounding resources. He is not simply content to fall into a routine or to let his disability take over his life. He is constantly changing and evolving, making adaptations and pursuing his life ambitions. James's wife commented that many people with health problems are quickly overwhelmed by melancholy whereas James is more accepting and more focused on what he needs to do. He wishes for an MS cure but plans and lives life as though it will never come.

There is also the advantage of having extensive training and experience in psychiatry—a field that naturally lends itself to gaining self-insight and modifying destructive paradigms. He is very aware of where he comes from and how that molds who he is today. Perhaps his tumultuous early childhood and strict parents prepared him to deal with the real-world difficulties he faces now. He may have learned subtle lessons about how to adapt to new environments and build new relationships. His father's alcoholism and emotional lability may have prepared him for the fluctuations and exacerbations he would later face with MS. Alcoholism is just a different kind of relapsing remitting disease, so James came into MS with extensive experience. Disadvantages can turn into advantages in the right setting.

We are all in some ways influenced in who we are because of our past. Our struggle then becomes how we deal with who we are because of our past, and we get past that. We get past those patterns.

Part of psychiatry is about reprogramming self-destructive habits and behaviors. The obvious examples are eating disorders, drug abuse, self-injury, and suicide. However, common problems such as depression and social anxiety also have significant ties to malignant behavior routines. I do not know if it is innate or planned, but James seems to have a handle on not only what he says and does but also on what he thinks and feels. Although he presents himself modestly, he has a remarkable self-confidence, perhaps stemming from a long history of achievement and overcoming obstacles. He treats other people well even when he has a run of bad luck...even when he is having a rough day…even when he is in physical pain… even when the world seems to conspire against him.

James also has superb judgment when making big decisions in life. He knows when to be aggressive and when to be passive. Sometimes, being resilient means never giving up and leaving no stone unturned. Other times, it requires adjustment and acceptance. James always seems to push and pull with exactly the right force. Talking to him and hearing his story makes me feel good about our society. Surely, people among us with serious health conditions are more productive and live a higher quality of life than in any time in history.

I do not know what the future holds for James. He and I are both young men, and I would like to believe that we will both witness a revolution of neuro-regenerative treatment. Conceivably, future technologies will make his current trials and tribulations disappear. Either way, I am certain he will continue to do amazing things.

CHAPTER FOUR REFERENCES

1. Meulenbeld GJ. Introduction. A History of Indian Medical Literature. Netherlands, n.p, 1999.
2. Tremlett H, Paty D, Devonshire V. Disability progression in multiple sclerosis is slower than previously reported. Neurology 2006 Jan 24;66(2):172-7.
3. Bakhuraysah MM, Siatskas C, Petratos C. Hematopoietic stem cell transplantation for multiple sclerosis: is it a clinical reality? Stem Cell Res Ther 2016;7:12.
4. Muraro PA, Douek DC, Packer A, et al. Thymic output generates a new and diverse TCR repertoire after autologous stem cell transplantation in multiple sclerosis patients. J Exp Med 2005;201(5):805-816.
5. Burt RK, Balabanov R, Han X, Sharrack B, Morgan A, Quigley K, Yaung K, Helenowski IB, Jovanovic B, Spahovic D, Arnautovic I, Lee DC, Benefield BC, Futterer S, Oliveira MC, Burman J. Association of nonmyeloablative hematopoietic stem cell transplantation with neurological disability in patients with relapsing-remitting multiple sclerosis. JAMA 2015 Jan 20;313(3):275-84.
6. Orenstein BW. Surprise Remission for Woman Diagnosed With MS and Breast Cancer. Everyday Health 2015. Available at http://www.everydayhealth.com/multiple-sclerosis/living-with/surprise-remission-woman-diagnosed-with-ms-breast-cancer/
7. Burt RK, Loh Y, Cohen B, et al. Autologous non-myeloablative haemopoietic stem cell transplantation in relapsing-remitting multiple sclerosis: a phase I/II study. Lancet Neurol. 2009;8(3):244-253.
8. Loh Y, Oyama Y, Statkute L, et al. Development of a secondary autoimmune disorder after hematopoietic stem cell

transplantation for autoimmune diseases: role of conditioning regimen used. Blood 2007;109(6):2643-548.

9. Nash RA, Hutton GJ. High-dose immunosuppressive therapy and autologous Hematopoietic Cell Transplantation for Relapsing-Remitting Multiple Sclerosis (HALT-MS): a 3-year interim report. *JAMA Neurol* 2015 Feb; 72(2): 159–169.

10. Marriage, divorce and adoption statistics (series FM2): Divorces, 1985–1998: sex and age at marriage. Orgainisation. Statbase Dataset Office for National Statistics 2010

11. Stenager E, Stenager EN, Knudsen L, et al. Multiple sclerosis: the impact on family and social life. Acta Psychiatr Belg 94:165–174.

12. Clarke L. Socio-demographic predictors of divorce. Family Policy Studies Centre and London School of Hygiene and Tropical Medicine 1998;Ann Berrington Department of Social Statistics, University of Southampton.

13. Torvik FA, Røysamb E, Gustavson K, Idstad M, Tambs K. Discordant and Concordant Alcohol Use in Spouses as Predictors of Marital Dissolution in the General Population: Results from the Hunt Study. Alcoholism clinical & experimental research 2013;May;37(5):877-84.

14. Kalmijn M, De Graaf PM , Janssen JPG. Intermarriage and the risk of divorce in the Netherlands: The effects of differences in religion and in nationality, 1974–94. *Popul Stud (Camb)* 2005 Mar;59(1):71-85.

15. Coles A, Deans J, Compston A. Multiple sclerosis treatment trial precipitates divorce. J Neurol Neurosurg Psychiatry 2001;70:135.

16. Fred Hutchinson Cancer Research Center. "Men Leave: Separation And Divorce Far More Common When The Wife Is The Patient." ScienceDaily. ScienceDaily, 10 November 2009.

CHAPTER 5:
THE PSYCHOLOGY
OF RESILIENCE

"Never forget what you are, for surely the world will not.
Make it your strength. Then it can never be your weakness.
Armour yourself in it, and it will never be used to hurt you."
—Tyrion Lannister in *A Game of Thrones* by George R.R. Martin

ONE OF MY friends is a neuromuscular disease expert, and he told me something very interesting. He has many patients with either amyotrophic lateral sclerosis (ALS) or myasthenia gravis (MG), both well-known neuromuscular diseases. ALS, the disease Stephen Hawking had, causes progressive degeneration of the motor neurons throughout the body, leading to gradual loss of muscle strength, speech, swallowing, and even breathing function. It is a horrible disease, and patients typically worsen relentlessly, suffering significant deterioration even a few years after diagnosis. My grandfather died of ALS, and his primary symptom was respiratory failure. In the end, he required continuous oxygen, and he was short of breath after taking a few steps with a walker. Myasthenia gravis, by contrast, is an autoimmune disease where the immune system attacks the neuromuscular junction. Although this is a serious condition, many patients do quite well with treatment, but they commonly have fluctuations of symptoms from day to day or even throughout the day.

Here is the interesting part: My colleague has noticed patients with ALS are almost always much happier and calmer than patients with myasthenia. Although receiving a diagnosis of ALS is devastating, once patients get over the initial shock, they are often accepting of their new condition and learn to adapt to their disabilities as they develop. My experience with ALS corroborates this as well; even as I disclose the diagnosis and prognosis, many of my patients are surprisingly calm and accepting. Myasthenia patients, on the other hand, are often anxious about new or fluctuating symptoms. They have periods of worsening and improvement. They have good days and bad days. When you know what it is like to feel good, feeling bad is more noticeable. ALS patients are used to having a disability and expect to get worse. It is in some ways easier to have ALS than it is to have myasthenia. With ALS, you do not have to look out for new symptoms or think about medication regimen changes.

MS's variability makes it much more comparable to myasthenia than to ALS. If you have MS and you are doing well, you worry about being in a wheelchair someday. If you have MS and you are significantly disabled, you wonder why other people with the same disease are doing so well, and you think about what you can do to get better. This is one of the great challenges of having a highly variable and unpredictable disease of unknown cause with no known cure. It is psychological torture.

Because of this, MS presents a tremendous challenge to the psyche and requires robust cognitive resources. As we have seen with Dr. Emily Spitz and Dr. James Bhat, resilience can make the difference between allowing an illness to destroy you and living a fulfilling life. To this effect, psychological resilience is the capacity to withstand and recover from threats to one's stability, vitality, development, and effectiveness as a person. The stress–diathesis model shown below conceptualizes how resilient individuals are more resistant to negative experiences and environments:

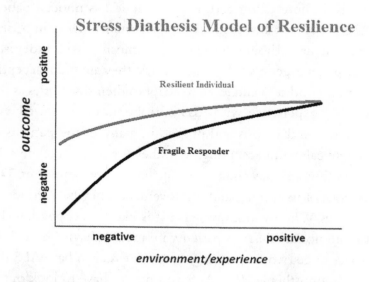

Figure 1: The Stress-Diathesis Model of Resilience; edited from the Wikimedia Commons

Due to the importance of characteristics of resilience in so many facets of life for such a diversity of circumstances, psychologists and psychiatrists have sought to better understand it and to foster it in their patients. Luckily, there is strong evidence resilience can be learned and improved over time[1], though developing it is perhaps more art than science. In seeking to better understand the psychology of resilience, I researched various schools of psychology and how they relate to resilience. I also interviewed Dr. Rex Beaber, a clinical psychologist who also happens to be my father. He has extensive experience in treating both general psychological conditions and medical patients with psychological comorbidities. He has also worked for the Los Angeles Police Department doing psychological evaluations on those arrested for murder. His comments are in italics throughout this chapter.

From the perspective of a psychologist, resilience is essentially a personality trait that facilitates adaptive and constructive responses to adversity. One aspect of resilience is affective or emotional. The resilient individual does not respond to adversity with paralyzing anxiety or disabling depression. In the resilient individual, their emotional response to adversity is attenuated and controlled. A second aspect of resilience is cognitive. The resilient individual is more likely to view adversity and its circumstances as a problem to solve. They understand that the circumstances of adversity are often beyond complete resolution, and rather than entering a state of despair and pessimism, they attempt to find some way to reduce their pain and suffering or the magnitude of the functional consequences of the adversity. An important distinguishing characteristic of the resilient individual, which is in marked contrast to the fragile responder, is that the resilient individual sees adversity in terms of a group of small, potentially solvable problems. The fragile responder, by focusing on the "big picture," is simply overwhelmed by tragic life events. Most importantly, the resilient responder knows when persistence might work but is also adept at knowing when to give up and conserve personal resources for another day or another problem. The power of lowering personal expectations when one has disabling adversity cannot be overstated.

COGNITIVE PSYCHOLOGY

My father alludes to the cognitive school of psychology as a way to approach resilience. This is essentially trying to understand resilience in terms of cognitive processes such as attention, thinking, memory, problem solving, and subconscious biases. You can also think of it as facing a tragedy in life in the same way you would face a technical task such as organizing a business or planning a social event. You set aside the emotional aspect and focus on the logistics of a practical approach. This includes understanding the problem, specifying goals, and taking reasonable action. In this way, resilience is more of a process than a trait.

Even the initial approach to a problem varies tremendously from person to person[2]. When I diagnose people with MS, some break down in tears while others are remarkably nonchalant. Sometimes, this nonchalance is because of naiveté or overconfidence, but it is usually because some people are simply comfortable being diagnosed with a chronic illness. They accept it as part of life. That being said, nothing is inherently wrong with being emotional so long as you can keep things under control. The goal is to experience emotions while maintaining the ability to cope and thrive. Amongst those that are initially overwhelmed, some are quick to adapt to the diagnosis. Some who are less emotional up-front falter in the long run. How we talk to ourselves about our current circumstances has a significant impact on our well-being and ability to cope with stressors. Our emotions are inextricably tied to our mindset because the emotional state is influenced by our thoughts, and our thoughts are influenced by our emotional state. When we have negative cognitive biases, we are more likely to be anxious, fearful, and pessimistic in response to events in life[3]. As Shakespeare's Hamlet says, "There is nothing either good or bad, but thinking makes it so." Furthermore, when our mood is depressed or anxious, our cognitive function deteriorates[4]. The result is a vicious cycle in what my father calls the "fragile responder." The individual is emotionally distraught and too overwhelmed to take corrective action. This failure to act further worsens her condition and emotional state.

I once consulted with a patient who had been suffering from post-concussive syndrome. The head injury was relatively mild, but for months afterwards, she languished with headaches, dizziness, lethargy, and various cognitive problems. She had been off work and was living with her relatives. She restricted herself to only the most basic activities, believing her brain needed rest and any significant activity would worsen her condition. She became despondent and dependent on others, thinking she would never return to her prior life. I reassured her she had no serious brain injury and that gradually resuming her normal activities would actually help her recover. In the next several weeks, she made excellent progress, returning to work and resuming a normal social life. I really did nothing for her except identify and challenge the negative thought patterns which were more harmful than the concussion itself.

I had another patient—let us call her Maria—with progressive MS who could barely walk with a walker and was slowly declining. Maria had convinced herself that if she could no longer walk, life would not be worth living, and she would commit suicide. She pursued a series of treatments and an aggressive rehab program, determined to maintain her walking ability. Despite all this, her progression continued. Although the decline was slow, she eventually reached a point where she could no longer walk. For a brief moment, she fell into the deepest despair, but her daughter convinced her it did not matter whether or not she could walk. She had spent the last several years in a wheelchair most of the time, and she realized she could still do everything she wanted to do. She could read, spend time with her family, and pursue various hobbies. Suddenly, she was happier than she had been in years. Her fear of losing the ability to walk was more upsetting than actually losing the ability to walk. These stories remind us that belief is just as important as reality.

The core idea is that behind every disabling emotion is a destructive idea or concept, which if rooted out and attacked, can result in improved affect and mood. The idea, for example, that "If I can't walk normally, it would be catastrophic" fosters depression and hopelessness. The slight change to "If I can't walk normally, it will make my life more difficult and inconvenient, but there are still many pleasures that are open to me" leads to a completely different emotional response.

When Maria changed her attitude towards disability, it did not make her less ambitious or reduce her self-care. She was still interested in seeking the best medical treatment, but she developed a more comprehensive approach. She focused more on lifestyle changes and adaptations. She learned to become less dependent on walking and to work around her disability to live a happy life. When she shifted her thinking patterns, everything became easier. The power of negative thinking comes naturally to people with MS and other neurological diseases, but it can affect all of us. Even a completely healthy person can destroy herself with hypochondriasis.

I have a distinctive memory of one of my more challenging cases that ended with a paradoxical twist. At the time, I was a faculty member of the UCLA Medical Center working with primary care physicians. A patient—we'll call her Margo—was referred to me by her primary care physician because she sought repeated medical testing for various cancers after having subjective symptoms that were relatively mild and non-specific. Even a cursory psychological examination revealed signs of a mixed affective disorder with elements of both depression and anxiety with a prominent obsession with cancer dating back to the death of her mother from cervical cancer.

Margo was a middle-aged woman trapped in a loveless marriage with a husband that had emotionally abandoned her due to her cancer phobia long ago. My two-year marathon attempt to give her some kind of psychic relief was an abysmal failure. Psychotropic intervention with anti-anxiety medication and anti-depressants did little. Cognitive approaches focusing on understanding cancer risk had no effect, albeit to make her obsession more technical. Psychodynamic approaches focusing on the significance of losing her mother to cancer during late childhood resulted in insight, a cathartic rainstorm of tears, but no reduction in dysphoria. My emotionally supportive efforts were appreciated but useless, and even a stint at hypnosis had no impact.

Finally after two years of psychotherapy, our treatment relationship ended when my career led me to another institution. Several years later, I returned to UCLA to visit faculty friends. To my surprise, there was Margo patiently waiting for her annual check-up. We talked, and I was shocked by her presentation. Her mood was upbeat; she laughed with some spontaneity; she didn't utter a word about cancer; and, she reported that her relationship with her husband was positively revived. While delighted by her progress, I was chagrined that someone else's technique succeeded where my efforts had failed. I queried: "What has produced this marked change in your mood?" A wry smile crossed her face as she explained: "Doctor, shortly after you left, I was diagnosed with cervical cancer." This was the transformative event. No longer fighting a ghost and having seen the face of the monster, she was liberated from her daunting fear.

RATIONAL EMOTIVE BEHAVIORAL THERAPY (REBT)

Margo's thinking about cancer changed dramatically, but we would all like to be able to change our thinking without years of therapy and fortuitous circumstances. Some psychologists have pushed us to directly confront and change our thinking in an analytical and systematic way. Dr. Albert Ellis established a style of therapy founded on this very idea which he called rational emotive behavioral therapy (REBT). The premise of REBT is that many emotional disturbances are founded on irrational thoughts. Margo's story above is an obvious example as she had an unjustified fear of cancer and unreasonable ideas about what a cancer diagnosis would mean to her. Not all of us are quite so neurotic, but we all have a bit of Margo within us. We fear things that are improbable or which would not be so bad if they came to fruition. We falsely imagine life would not be worth living if things did not go our way. Ellis believes we can train ourselves to think rationally by confronting and challenging our beliefs.

One strategy Ellis recommends is to break down responses to troubling circumstances into, "A," "B," and "C"[5, page 14]. These letters stand for Adversity, Beliefs, and Consequences. Let us take, for example, the story of the neurologist Dr. Emily Spitz (Chapter Two) when she was in the midst of her major relapse. She found herself clumsy, imbalanced, and dependent on her husband and mother. The attack turned her entire lifestyle upside down and forced her to stop working. When you are under such tremendous stress, there is a tendency to ignore beliefs and to make a direct jump from adversity to consequences such as this:

A: I am having a major MS flare, and I can hardly walk.
C: I cannot practice medicine or live a normal life.

However, intermediate between A and C is an intervening belief (B) that leads to a perception of consequences. When we add in the B, it becomes clearer:

A: I am having a major MS flare, and I can hardly walk.

B: I fear I will never recover, and I do not have confidence in my ability to adapt to a disability to continue to work and to face the daily challenges of living. I also think about how people will see me as disabled and treat me differently.

C: I cannot practice medicine or live a normal life.

Facing a severe MS relapse, it is understandable she would think along these lines. Going from highly-functional to significantly impaired in a matter of days would shake any sensible person's confidence. However, the belief listed above is fundamentally irrational. It is an emotional reaction not founded in reality. If we change the belief, we can change the perceived consequences as follows:

A: I am having a major MS flare, and I can hardly walk.

B: Although I fear I will never recover, it is likely I will improve at least somewhat. Even if I do not, I will become accustomed to any disabilities over time, and I will learn to adapt. My family is very supportive and willing to help. If other people view me differently, it really does not matter to me.

C: Although this flare is very inconvenient and distressing, I will still be able to practice medicine and live a happy and fulfilling life.

Even before she recovered from her flare, Emily Spitz learned to change her thinking, and while she was in the hospital, her emotional state improved dramatically. Emotions are not just the result of events in our lives; they result from our interpretations of these events. These interpretations are often clouded, biased, and floridly irrational. It is not enough to look for distractions or hope for the best. We must look to make deep-seated philosophical changes if we want to be more resilient in the long run.

As I explained in the opening chapter, MS is a disease that often produces a tremendous amount of anxiety. It is aimless, arbitrary, and unpredictable. People often imagine the worst, and even when they are doing well, they may be bogged down by a hundred invisible symptoms. A natural fear of the future comes with MS. Because of this, people with MS often irrationally see things as worse than they really are. Even when they are doing well, some of my patients view their situation as "horrible," "awful," and "catastrophic." Albert Ellis calls this "horribilizing," "awfulizing," and "catastrophizing." People often demand things "must" be different than they are. Ellis calls this "musturbation"[5, page 65].

I am not trying to downplay the significance of MS symptoms. I would never tell a patient they do not have pain or that they are exaggerating their grievances. However, I do think many people irrationally underestimate their ability to be resilient and adapt to change. The problem with "catastrophizing" is not only that it is emotionally distressing, but it also encourages us to look for short-sighted and temporary solutions. You might quit a stressful job, abandon a relationship, or take a drug to treat a symptom. These may be reasonable actions in some cases, but they may be detrimental in the long term or could distract us from looking to change our mindset. Whether or not you have MS, it is toxic to believe things "should," "must," or "ought" to work out a certain way. This "shoulding," "musting," and "oughting" is a backwards way of thinking. Life guarantees us nothing; the world delivers, and we must react to it, not the other way around. Try to think of fear, anxiety, and other distressing thoughts as what they really are: neurophysiologic processes in the physical brain subject to modification through various techniques[6].

I had a patient with MS who came to me in great distress. She was in her early sixties, and although her physical problems were fairly mild, she bemoaned that her gait was declining gradually. I examined her and found subtle gait impairment, and I diagnosed her with secondary progressive MS. Her problems were slight and would not be obvious to a casual observer, but she was otherwise fit and vibrant, so losing function was understandably troubling to her. I followed her for the next few years, and we tried various treatments. She visited me every three months, and each encounter was remarkably similar: She would complain that she had dramatically deteriorated since the prior visit, and she was visibly uneasy to the point of speaking rapidly with a quavering voice. On examination, she appeared to be approximately stable, but we would review treatment options and make changes. After several such visits, each beginning with grievances about her significant decline in the last few months, I confronted her about the issue. We came to an understanding that she was not truly losing function and was actually able to do everything she could do before. She agreed to seek treatment for her anxiety, and she attempted to change her feeling that MS was an unacceptable fate. Since that time, her mood has dramatically improved, and she considers herself lucky to have done so well despite a long history of the disease.

PERSPECTIVE

Sometimes, it helps to have a little perspective. When I was a medical student, I remember my experience on a psychiatry rotation covering the inpatient unit. Many of our patients were schizophrenics with florid psychosis. Others had bipolar disorder and were in a fulminant manic phase. They were severely impaired, requiring constant observation and drugs to control their behavior. We would also get a few depressed patients who were admitted after contemplating suicide. They would often see the other patients and consider themselves extremely fortunate by comparison. This sense of perspective was just as helpful as medications and therapy, and we would often discharge them within a few days. It is helpful to think about your life in the broad context of human existence. Perhaps medicine is the best profession in that we as physicians are constantly surrounded by the less fortunate.

Even if you are not ruminating about your misfortune, it is easy to criticize your own abilities and talents as we live in a very achievement-oriented society. When people are diagnosed with MS, they are sometimes too self-critical, and they may sabotage their own self-confidence. I had a patient give up driving after an ophthalmologist said her optic nerves looked abnormal even though her visual function was excellent. I have had patients who are afraid to have children because they question their abilities as a parent. In reality, these people would probably make for very conscientious parents because they care enough to question their own abilities. I have had many patients ask me if they will be able to succeed in their career when they are already successful. Ellis calls this style of thinking "self-downing"[5, page 89].

It can be very troubling when someone with MS compares herself to people who are completely healthy. We are social beings, and we sometimes think in a competitive and hierarchical way. This is natural but not always useful. We should judge ourselves in the context of our own unique situation. When James Bhat is struggling to do something he could have done easily ten years ago, it makes little sense to compare the feat to what it was ten years ago. It is a greater feat. When Dr. Bhat does his morning routine and goes to work, he is expertly performing a series of coordinated and practiced movements, all requiring maneuvers to compensate for his physical limitations. He is like a trapeze artist in a circus show or a shortstop fielding a one-hopper. If I were magically transported into his body, I could never do what he does. I would cut myself shaving, trip over things, and spill my drink.

It is also harmful to look to others to provide a sense of personal value. Physical health, career success, and loving relationships are variable, relative, and subjective. Even billionaires and elite athletes often find themselves in the offices of psychiatrists. It is better to like yourself just for being who you are. People can give you an extrinsic self-worth, but only you can give yourself an intrinsic self-worth. Seeking the approval of others will only lead to temporary happiness. Whereas downplaying what others think of you and focusing on your own desires and aspirations encourages you to pursue what Ellis calls a "long range hedonism"[5, page 107]. Life on Earth is far from nirvana, but we can find great joy if we look for it. Focusing on yourself also helps you to be more active and less passive because you are always more in control of yourself than you are of others.

People like Ellis also criticize an over-emphasis on past events. Even if early childhood traumas and other negative life events shape who we are, they should not thwart our personal progress. Ninety percent of people will experience at least one major trauma in life[7], so we must learn to live with a history of trauma. One problem with Freud's psychoanalytic method is that it fosters an obsession with the past. Psychodynamic therapies often focus on insight and catharsis as the catalyst to change. Sometimes, it is helpful to understand the past as an explanation for our irrational thinking. However, insight into the source of a problem alone does not result in effective behavioral change. More proactive coping strategies, whether they be behavioral or cognitive, are necessary. Therapies such as rational emotive behavioral therapy (REBT) along with cognitive-behavioral therapy (CBT), dialectical behavioral therapy (DBT), and acceptance and commitment therapy (ACT) focus not only on self-understanding but also on making concrete changes towards value-driven behavior to decrease symptoms and increase well-being. Let us say I am afraid of flying. It does not really matter why I have this fear so long as I can recognize that it is irrational and work on changing my underlying beliefs.

Rational emotive behavioral therapy is about rational thinking and practical moderation. It is valuable to be concerned, but it is harmful to be over-concerned and paralyzed by fear. We must remember frustration is not the same as catastrophe. When I think about Dr. James Bhat, it seems so obvious that one of his big advantages is he is so calm and rational. He does not think to himself, "I can hardly walk! This is terrible!" He thinks, "It is inconvenient that MS has limited my mobility, so I will have to do things differently. I will hire a driver to get to work. I will use a baby monitor to call patients into my office." He is not blindly optimistic and Pollyanna-ish—just stoically rational. He accepts that setbacks and annoyances are an expected part of life, especially for someone with MS. Also, James has what psychologists call universal self-acceptance. He is not just a psychiatrist, a husband, and a father. He is not just someone with MS. He is the one and only James Bhat with his own personality, desires, and idiosyncrasies, and he likes himself for who he is. Nothing and no one can take this away from him.

ASSIMILATIVE AND ACCOMMODATIVE COPING

James is a person who does not let changes bother him excessively. This comes very naturally to him, but for the rest of us, it is an uphill battle. When we face a challenge in life, there are two fundamental approaches: acceptance and resistance. We can try to change the problem, or we can change ourselves so our outlook and goals align with our new reality. Psychologists have called these approaches "assimilative" and "accommodative" coping responses respectively[8]. When we have a problem which is fundamentally solvable, it makes sense to refuse to accept it and to maintain our existing goals and aspirations. When a problem is fundamentally less solvable through our own actions, we must be more accommodating, or it would be impossible to move on with life. It feels so natural to fight vigorously, but in the real world, some element of both coping responses is appropriate.

Let us say, for example, I am attempting to lose weight. I might take an assimilative approach and start a diet and exercise plan, but I have to at least temporarily accept I am overweight. I even must accept the possibility of setbacks or failure in the long run. If I can be accommodating in this way, I am more likely to have the confidence and positivity needed to succeed. Also, I am more likely to be happy with myself if I fail or achieve partial success. With this flexible approach and inner acceptance, I am less likely to fall off the wagon after a stumbling block. With MS, you might accept that you have a disease along with the downsides and uncertainties that come with it, but at the same time, you can continue to enjoy life and pursue the goals which are still feasible. It takes good judgment to know when we must resist and when we must acquiesce. We must know when to be rigid and when to be flexible. James knows that he cannot run marathons, but he can still practice psychiatry.

To change the natural inclination towards an overly assimilative coping response, therapists have attempted what is known as "cognitive bias modification"[9]. This is where emotional responses to a stimulus are modified in a controlled setting. For instance, someone with claustrophobia might ride an elevator with a therapist while receiving comforting encouragement. They might ask a patient with anger management problems to reenact an upsetting interaction in a friendly and non-confrontational manner. A person with MS might imagine themselves experiencing a relapse and taking the appropriate action without excessive worry. They might picture themselves with the disability they most fear while visualizing that they can adapt and live happily.

On the other side of the coin, I have had many patients who have an excessively accommodative coping response. I have seen people wait until they are in a wheelchair before even seeing a doctor. I have seen countless others ravage their bodies with the American diet and a sedentary lifestyle. One of my patients refused to take his epilepsy medication and had a seizure while driving, killing his mother in the passenger seat. Needless to say, this blithe attitude is not the goal. It is extremely important to be vigilant, proactive, and self-advocating. A comprehensive and balanced approach incorporates both accommodative and assimilative coping styles.

POSITIVE PSYCHOLOGY

One of the general criticisms of the field of psychology is it has historically been geared towards treating the sick. Those with depression, bipolar disorder, schizophrenia, and other disabling illnesses have been the focus of the field for most of its existence. In 1998, Martin Seligman became the president of the American Psychological Association, and he vowed to encourage the field to improve the lives of ordinary people without specific psychological disorders[10]. It is one thing to make a miserable person content or a psychotic person reasonable. It is an entirely different thing to help an ordinary person to flourish, thrive, and live to her fullest potential. The latter is in the realm of the field that we now know as positive psychology.

Needless to say, becoming happier is an important part of resilience. It is easier for happier people to have the realistic optimism described in Chapter Three. Positive emotions help people forge stronger relationships. There are numerous health benefits as well. Happier people have a lower resting heart rate and a milder elevation of fibrinogen in response to stress[11]. Fibrinogen is an inflammatory marker in the blood which correlates with blood viscosity and risk of heart disease[12]. Happy people also tend to live longer[13]. A study of elderly nuns found that those who expressed the most positive emotions earlier in life lived up to ten years longer than the group of nuns who had the least positive emotions[14].

Extremely happy people are not necessarily better looking, more religious, wealthier, or more fit than you and me. They do not always experience more good fortune and less bad fortune, but they are usually more social and often have a rich repertoire of friends. Also, they tend to be in romantic relationships, and they generally have a positive view of themselves and their circumstances[15]. Indeed, good mental health comes from having a positive interpretation of one's own traits and subjective experiences in the world. Happiness is not simply a genetic inborn trait. Research suggests that doing the following may increase your happiness:

1. Eat abundant whole fruits and vegetables[16, 17]
2. Become financially secure[18, 19]-though research suggests you may not gain additional happiness beyond a salary of $75,000 US dollars per year
3. Develop a strong social network[19, 20]
4. Find a job/career you enjoy[19]
5. Get married[21], especially to a happy person[22]
6. Spend time with happy people[23]
7. Exercise[24, 25]

Unfortunately, high intelligence and a high level of education do not seem to increase happiness[26]. The effect of having children on happiness is unclear as children increase stress but provide a source of greater meaning[27-30]. Poor health does tend to contribute to lower subjective happiness[31], though the effect is more modest than we would expect. Generally, both positive and negative events have less of an effect on happiness than people anticipate. Positive events such as getting a promotion usually only produce brief happiness, and negative events such as failing an examination yield only a temporary reduction in happiness[32].

Martin Seligman describes three forms of happiness[33] which he calls pleasure, engagement, and meaning. He describes the pleasant life as a life full of gratifying experiences and positive emotions. Eating ice cream, laughing at a joke, and exercising are all hedonistic experiences which contribute to a happy life. They cause a clear and palpable form of happiness. The only problem with the pleasurable life is we become habituated to pleasurable experiences, and they make us less happy over time. Also, there is a significant genetic component to hedonic pleasure[34], and it is only partly modifiable. For these reasons, Seligman believes simple pleasure is the least important of the three contributions to happiness.

Engagement is the sensation of immersion in an activity or experience. You may be an engineer crafting an intricate contraption or a chef cooking an exquisite specialty. You may be playing a game of basketball or chess. You are engrossed and focused, paying little attention to distractions and thinking about nothing but the task at hand. Time becomes irrelevant and passes quickly. The activity becomes an end unto itself. It does not matter if a chef delivers the finished plate to an eager patron or throws it in a dumpster; there would still be enjoyment in cooking it.

The experience of total engagement and absorption into a pursuit has been called "flow." This is a state of intense concentration without apprehension. You feel you are being challenged but that your abilities are well suited to meet the current demands. You are neither stressed nor bored. In his book, *Flow: The Psychology of Optimal Experience*, the positive psychologist Mihaly Csikszentmihalyi describes the phenomenon:

"The mystique of rock climbing is climbing; you get to the top of a rock glad it's over but really wish it would go on forever. The justification of climbing is climbing, like the justification of poetry is writing; you don't conquer anything except things in yourself.... The purpose of flow is to keep on flowing, not looking for a peak or utopia but staying in the flow."[35]

We all experience flow and engagement at times. I actually remember my very first night on call back in 2009. Objectively, it was a miserable experience. I was up all night admitting patients, and I was anxiously making clinical decisions while learning the electronic medical record and the hospital system at the same time. I still recall a critically ill septic patient whom I was admitting to the intensive care unit. I was frazzled, trying to keep this poor young man alive. However, I was so pumped up and focused that I hardly had a chance to feel tired, and before I knew it, my call was over. I remember leaving the hospital energized and satisfied. Strangely, taking these calls became harder over time even though I was more experienced because I became much less engaged. The incredible energy and singular focus I had at the beginning of my internship would be impossible to replicate.

The third aspect of a happy life is finding a sense of meaning or purpose. Even a mirthless and tedious task can be fulfilling if we believe it contributes to a greater good or ultimate goal. We are constantly seeking a sense of meaning in life. We take jobs for lower pay because we believe they are altruistic. We make countless sacrifices for our children for nothing in return except the satisfaction of giving them a better life. We volunteer for religious and public aid organizations in our sparse free time.

Seligman has refined his ideas about positive psychology, and he also has studied the importance of relationships and achievements in living a happy life. He adds these concepts to the three forms of happiness above to form the acronym PERMA[36]:

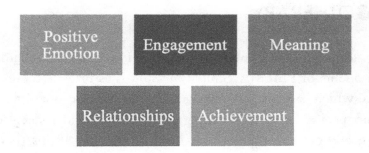

Humans are intrinsically a social species, and it is very difficult to be maximally content and productive without strong interpersonal relationships. We are also highly achievement oriented, and much of our sense of self-confidence and purpose comes from achieving goals. This can work against us if we are constantly comparing ourselves to others, but it can also work for us. I believe people with MS can use the principles of PERMA to be both happier and more resilient. Do things you enjoy more often. Pursue a hobby, interest, or career which engages you. Search for a long-term grand purpose you find meaningful. Strengthen important relationships in your life. Try to achieve everything you can, even if you must do so in the face of limitations. When you are happier, it will be easier to get your life back together in the face of a relapse, and you will more naturally adjust to new disabilities and to MS symptoms.

In the face of positivity, there will always be antagonistic negative thoughts trying to bring you down. Because of this, Seligman recapitulates the wisdom of rational emotive behavioral therapy. As he says, you should be "treating the catastrophic thoughts as if they were uttered by an external person whose mission is to make your life miserable, and then marshaling evidence against the thoughts"[37]. It is always more valuable to think about what you can control than what you cannot control. Luckily, there is almost always something within PERMA you can influence and optimize.

LOGOTHERAPY

The meaningful life is perhaps the most important of Seligman's components of PERMA. Simple pleasure is as brief as the experience which causes it, and engagement depends on our ability to pursue specific activities. Meaning, on the other hand, is deep, long lasting, and not easily taken away from us. Because of this, there is an entire field of psychology dedicated to it. Logotherapy was invented by the great German psychiatrist and author Viktor Frankl. In his famous book, *Man's Search for Meaning*, Frankl describes his experiences as a Jewish captive during the Holocaust as he moves through a series of Nazi work camps prior to and during World War II. He chronicles the nightmare of the camps in vivid and harrowing detail, and he personally suffers a series of abuses that disturb the reader and tear at the human soul. One thing that helps him to fight through the ordeal and to maintain hope is his ability to find meaning within his suffering.

Logotherapy is a "will to meaning,"[38, pg. 99] the idea that the primary source of satisfaction and mental stability is finding a meaning or purpose to one's life. You must have an overarching goal to inspire yourself to feel good about minor victories and to persevere in the worst of times. He contrasts this with what Alfred Adler called "striving to assert superiority" which is merely giving yourself value in comparison to other people. He also contrasts this with Sigmund Freud's "pleasure principle" which is simply the craving to appease basic desires. Meaning is deeply personal and constantly changing, and we can have multiple sources of meaning at once. When my children were born, I developed an incredible fascination with them while the importance of my friends and hobbies diminished. When I was younger, academic achievement meant much more to me than it does now, and as I grow older, I will need to find new and different sources of meaning.

Although meaning may change, it should be something which can robustly and consistently guide us for a period of time. It must not be something trivial or selfish. It should be grand, outward, and altruistic—something important to us we can take pride in. That being said, it does not have to be something that would result in widespread recognition such as running a successful business or discovering a great scientific breakthrough. It can be something as simple as being kind and bringing joy and happiness to strangers.

Princess Diana believed if she could give love to someone for one minute, it would be important and meaningful[39].

Of course, not everyone has the same privileges and opportunities as the Princess of Wales. During the Nazi regime, many Jews wondered if they would even survive. This is surely a natural thought to have, but Frankl thought of something different: "Has all this suffering, this dying around us, a meaning? For if not, then ultimately there is no meaning to survival"[38, pg. 115]. In other words, if there is no meaning to your life, you are dead already.

Logotherapy is best applied to what some call the tragic triad of life: pain, guilt, and death [38, pg. 137]. We must turn our pain into achievements; we must turn guilt into motivation to improve ourselves; we must turn fear of death into a call for action[38, pg. 138]. According to Frankl, many concentration camp prisoners would fall into a sort of existential abyss, losing all emotion and desire to continue the struggle to survive. They would effectively give up and succumb to starvation, illness, or violence. Frankl, however, struggled to find meaning in his suffering. He thought about his love for his estranged wife and visualized her smile. He longed to unleash logotherapy unto the world and to resume his career as a psychiatrist. He imagined his family members watching from the heavens and tried to act in a way which would make them proud. His captors could take away his possessions, his clothing, his family, and his career, but they could not change his attitude or his inner freedom. Even a man forced into the gas chambers chooses his final thoughts before his death.

There are different broad categories of meaning in life. One form of meaning is love and relationships with other people. Another form of meaning is achievement—some form of work, productivity, or opus magnus. Yet another form of meaning is seeking experiences in the world be they through travel, hobbies, or special events. The final form of meaning is through conflict and suffering.

This is the fulfillment of overcoming the greatest challenges we face in life or in turning tragedy into success[38 pg. 145-146].

Logotherapy is predicated on the notion that we have freedom to find meaning in what we do and what we experience—or at least in the stand we take when faced with a situation of unchangeable suffering, as with chronic disease. It is critically important that someone with a chronic and unrelenting disease learn that "everything can be taken from a man but one thing: the last of the human freedoms—to choose one's attitude in any given set of circumstances."[38] It is important to be cognizant of the fact that the search for meaning is such a dominating force in most people that they will construct meaning on their own, and this meaning will sometimes be dysfunctional and will operate unconsciously in a destructive manner. For example, many patients imagine their illness as a deserved punishment. Often, this kind of depressogenic thought process must be rooted out and destroyed by the therapist.

Aside from the dysfunctional thoughts mentioned by my father, having an underlying meaning in life helps to promote hardiness, the characteristic of resistance to life stresses. Those with the personality trait of hardiness tend to be committed to finding a purpose in life and have a strong sense of personal agency[40-42]. Meaning and hardiness predispose resilience whereas hopelessness and a loss of personal agency are associated with depression and are even linked to suicide. Where there is meaning, there is hope, and where there is hope, there is a reason to live and flourish.

Sometimes meaning comes naturally, but we can also construct it. In one study, Carolyn Schwartz and Meir Sendor had patients with MS call other patients with MS once a month for a year, instructing them to provide emotional support in any way they could. At the end of the study, the callers had themselves benefited and had greater confidence and self-esteem than the patients they were calling[43]. The meaning given to the callers proved more helpful than the support received by those being called. It is truly better to give than to receive.

Finding meaning is a personal endeavor, but the opportunities are endless. Forget for a moment about your weaknesses and your flaws. What is it that makes you great? What is it that makes you exceptional? Think about your greatest strengths, and attempt to exploit them to do something important to you. Develop a new talent. Volunteer for a charity. Create a great work of art or write a memoir. Become a mentor to a family member or a stranger. Pursue a religious or spiritual endeavor. The benefits will become self-evident as soon as you get started. A disease like MS often forces people to experience a change in identity. This can shake up your sense of self and make you feel helpless and dependent, causing a form of existential crisis. Try to use this kairotic moment to reevaluate yourself and look for new sources of meaning and purpose in life.

ACCEPTANCE AND COMMITMENT THERAPY (ACT)

When we focus on the meaning of our choices, it facilitates a deep understanding of our true life values. A modern and recently popularized school of psychology known as Acceptance and Commitment Therapy (ACT) encourages us to clarify these values explicitly and take action toward living in their service. What is most important to you, and how would you want people to remember you? What do you want written on your tombstone? These are not necessarily society's values or the values expected of us; rather, they are the principles, characteristics, and goals that appeal to you as an individual, uniquely and intuitively.

Try the following exercise: Think of eight core guiding ideas which will have the highest priority in your life. You can think of anything that comes to mind, but a few possibilities are in the table below.

Table of values

Achievement	Adventure	Altruism	Art
Dependability	Hobbies	Ethics	Fairness
Friendship	Free Time	Family	Travel
Independence	Influence	Integrity	Modesty
Intimacy	Popularity	Loyalty	Religion
Spirituality	Social Life	Fitness	Status
Connectedness	Honesty	Security	Wealth
Trustworthiness	Romance	Nature	Courage
Relaxation	Children	Sacrifice	Fun
Learning	Hard work	Beauty	Health
Respect	Golden Rule		

What do these values mean to you, and how do they apply to your life? What changes could you make to live in accordance with these ideas? In what areas are your behaviors incongruent with the person you want to be and what you want to achieve? When I was younger, I knew I wanted a family, but I was wholly focused on my studies and put little effort into dating. As I grew older, I learned to balance out my life and began to take dating quite seriously, as though it were a second career. We must not merely admire our values with empty smugness because they only have meaning if we put them into action. If I say I value honesty, but I am not honest, it is just theoretical. If I say I value hard work while lounging and filibustering, it means very little. You must commit to making changes and living in the spirit of your core beliefs[45] (hence the "commitment" part of ACT).

ACT also modifies traditional cognitive-behavioral therapy to encourage acceptance of undesirable thoughts and emotions[46]. In a process known as "cognitive fusion," we sometimes mistake our negative thoughts of anxiety and fear with reality. Changing how we think can be effective, but it sometimes feels unnatural and strained. It may be easier to hold our negative thoughts close to us, understand them, and place them in perspective. This gives us the psychological flexibility we need to face the ebbs and flows of a chronic disease like MS[47,48]. In fact, ACT has been used in resilience training in MS, showing benefits in mental health, depression, and stress levels[49]. It has also been used to manage MS pain[50].

To better understand ACT, I interviewed experts on the topic. One of them, Dr. John Forsyth, is a clinical psychologist, speaker, and author of several books including *The Mindfulness & Acceptance Workbook for Anxiety*. I asked him to summarize the key concepts and how they apply to MS and other chronic diseases.

The central idea of ACT is one of changing our relationship with the stuff we carry in the service of what matters to us. We struggle with what we think, feel, remember, and so on, having learned that painful thoughts and feelings must be changed in order to be happy and to live a vital life. This is a trap.

Science teaches us that the more you don't want a painful thought or emotion, the more you've got it. There's no healthy way not to think a thought without thinking it (try not thinking about a pink elephant, and you'll get what I mean). This struggle takes enormous effort, and all the time and energy focused on changing our thinking, our feeling, and what our bodies are doing is time, energy, and attention away from what we really care about. We swim in a sea of thoughts, and we soon start to trust and believe what we think, even if it doesn't serve us well in terms of the kind of life we wish to lead.

Culture feeds this too because it teaches us we should be happy, happy, happy. It teaches us that pain is a problem and a barrier to happiness, so you'd better do something about your pain in order to be happy. And with that, the trap door is slammed shut, and we are set up to struggle with the painful thoughts, feelings, and physical sensations we feel on the inside. And this just makes things worse in the long run. Our lives get smaller. The suffering gets bigger. Meanwhile, life is not getting lived, and for many, this is the worst pain of all.

ACT teaches us to be more flexible, learning to be kind and gentle with ourselves and what our mind and body offers us so that we have the space to choose to engage what we do care about, even if the mind protests—because it likely will. In short, we learn to let go of trying to influence what we have limited control over (thoughts, images, judgments, physical sensations or feelings that arise in our bodies and minds) and focus on what we do have control over—how we respond to what we think and feel and what we do with our mouths, hands, and feet.

We saw how Dr. James Bhat in the prior chapter was able to demonstrate incredible psychological flexibility, learning to adapt to his disabilities as they arose and always fighting to live the life he wanted. When your eye is on the prize (your true values and ambitions), it is easier to tread through turbulence.

When humans face pain, we tend to harden and narrow. We get small—like if a hungry lion walked into your living room, everything else around you would wash away, and all your attention would be focused on that lion. We narrow and life around us washes away. MS can be like that.

MS is not a choice. It happens. When the physical and psychological challenges arise with MS, it can feel like that hungry lion. There is so much life around you. You have things you want to do, hopes, dreams, and experiences that lift you up and bring meaning to your life. But when the MS lion rears its head, your life washes away, and it is so easy for all our energy to focus on the MS lion. But that is not what most people want. If one could just get rid of the MS lion, most people would, but MS doesn't work like that. So, the skillful trick is to learn to acknowledge the MS lion and then practice bringing your awareness to the things around you that you do want to nurture and engage—the things in your life that really matter to you. In a way, it's like bringing the MS lion along and no longer feeding it with your attention and precious energy and resources.

Athletes are taught that they must be flexible or else risk injury, and life is like that too. When pain and difficulty show up, we tend to narrow and get small. This would be fine if there was a real lion after us, but most of us don't have to face hungry lions day in and day out. But we do have to face our histories, all the stuff we carry, and the unpleasant stuff that our minds and bodies offer now and then. Here, we have a choice: we can feed the lion with our precious attention and energy, or we can acknowledge it, create space, stretch, and bring our awareness to what matters to us, lion or not.

And yes, MS may make it very hard to do what you used to do, but that doesn't mean you no longer care. You may need to practice being flexible. We had a man once in our ACT for MS workshop who valued play with his kids. This normally took the form of playing pickup basketball and running around the soccer field, but since he developed MS, these activities became hard for him to do. He was very sad about this and felt *like less of a dad. We then helped him step back and look at unhelpful thoughts that were keeping him stuck and helped him think more flexibly about what he could do to support his value of playtime with his kids. He then came up with other activities he could do with his kids, even with his MS—like swimming in a pool, playing board games, and developing a new hobby by getting the family a telescope to look at the moon and planets.*

MS is not a choice, but you have a choice in how you relate with the ups and downs that MS offers. This is where people have control, and ACT is really about learning skills, so you can make the most out of your life without letting MS control you.

You may protest that it is not so easy to prevent MS from taking over your life. Indeed, if you are suffering from neuropathic pain, it would be brusque to ask you to accept it and move on. Some symptoms of MS are unnerving, pervasive, and capable of shaking the psyche of the most resilient victim. To address this, I spoke with Dr. Melissa Fledderjohann, a clinical psychologist and director of pain management at San Mateo Medical Center in Northern California. She has had great success with an ACT-based multidisciplinary pain management approach. I asked her to explain how the ACT model applies to the management of chronic pain, and even though her focus is more on improving function than reducing pain, she reports optimistic results.

I use the following equation to teach the concepts of ACT:

Suffering = Pain x Resistance

This equation means that the more you resist pain, the more you tend to experience it, and this vicious cycle leads to suffering. Resistance in the medical model manifests as frequent and multiple doctor visits, second opinions, or unnecessary procedures and medications, all with the intention of trying to stop the pain. It is my goal to have my patients eliminate the suffering component of the equation and understand its opposite form: Wellbeing = Acceptance / Pain.

Acceptance is acknowledging pain and medical diagnoses while pursuing valued life activities in the presence of pain. It requires a willingness to remain in contact with the active experience, including both good and bad experiences. The ACT approach to pain involves two fundamental concepts. First, you must accept the aspects of pain that cannot change, including all the difficult thoughts, feelings, and bodily sensations that come with it. Second, acceptance allows patients the space to commit to acting in ways that make them feel vital and energized. ACT is not giving up hope for a better life; it is continuing to actively engage in meaningful behaviors which can lead to increased quality of life and pain reduction.

ACT has a technique called cognitive defusion which is the willingness to let go of attachment and over-identification with thoughts. When people are fused with thoughts, their identity becomes their beliefs. For example, "I'm medically ill; therefore, I am a sick person." Fusion becomes problematic because thoughts are believed as facts, and this serves to keep people stuck in patterns of thinking that lead to emotional suffering. Cognitive defusion is a tool that serves to disentangle people from their thoughts that cause suffering. The first step is to recognize that you are the observer of your thoughts, not the thoughts themselves. Freedom from unnecessary emotional suffering begins with a willingness to look at thoughts differently and let go of attachment to thoughts, especially those which are negative. One common exercise is to consider thoughts as though they are clouds in the sky or leaves floating down a stream.

Both Emily Spitz and James Bhat in Chapters Two and Four had strong identities outside of MS. Neither of them thought of themselves as defined by the disease, and this helped them to focus on other aspects of life. What they did fortuitously and intuitively can also be done purposefully and intentionally.

I had a patient—call her Jane—with a history of both childhood and adult trauma. In her mid-forties, she was suffering from chronic neck and back pain due to multiple herniated discs. Epidural injections and spinal surgery yielded minimal improvement, and she presented to our clinic with severe pain, anxiety, depression, and catastrophizing thoughts. Jane attended individual and group therapy, did mindfulness meditation, and walked four miles a day, several days a week. Over the course of a year, she lost twenty-five pounds, saw her psychiatric conditions improve along with her pain, successfully weaning off of her opioid medications.

I tell patients they are much more than their medical or mental health diagnoses and they can choose to step forward toward living life now in this moment. I help them through the grieving process that occurs with a diagnosis of chronic disease. Grieving means they have lived and that letting go is not the end but can be the beginning. They can live full and meaningful lives while still having medical and psychological problems, and they are not their diagnoses. They are much more than they believe.

THE AMERICAN PSYCHOLOGICAL ASSOCIATION

In practice, many of the principles I discussed in this chapter are used in combination depending upon your unique situation. If you find you have harmful patterns of thinking, focus on cognitive psychology or rational emotive behavioral therapy. If you are having difficulty with a new symptom or disability, try to gain perspective, and focus on accommodative coping. Use the principles of positive psychology even when you are feeling well, and always look for a grand purpose in life. The American Psychological Association summarizes some of these ideas and recommends ten ways to actively build resilience[44]:

1. **Form strong relationships with your family, friends, and community.** Be active in civic and religious organizations and pursue altruistic endeavors. Helping others and being part of a community will give you a sense of purpose and fulfillment.

2. **View big problems as solvable or adaptable.** Try not to think of new conflicts in life as catastrophic and permanent even if they carry very real consequences. Being diagnosed with MS or suffering an MS relapse is no trivial matter, but we can ameliorate many aspects of MS. Try to think about how things may improve in the future or how you can better adapt to present circumstances.

3. **Appreciate change as part of life.** Even if you cannot restore complete normalcy, realize that adapting to new challenges is part of the spice and excitement of life. Acceptance of changes such as newfound disability allows you to progress to the further steps of resilience.

4. **Make goals.** Think of a few things you would like to achieve, and create formal short-term goals. Be practical about what you can reasonably accomplish, and set out a written plan. Break down long-term goals into manageable smaller tasks.

5. **Take action.** Instead of ruminating on stressful situations or wallowing in despair, try to be proactive. Start doing something immediately to improve your situation.

6. **Improve yourself.** Look at your adversity as a way to rediscover and better yourself. If you have a limitation, try to learn a new skill to compensate for this. Strengthen your relationships with those who can help you while you are vulnerable and look for a silver lining.

7. **Think positively**. No matter how bad things get, remain confident in your ability to adapt, think on the fly, and solve problems. Know that you are a resilient person at heart, and trust yourself to make the best out of your circumstances.

8. **Maintain a healthy perspective.** When you are facing a problem which affects one aspect of life, try to look at the broader picture. Be thankful for the things you still have in life and avoid catastrophizing minor setbacks.

9. **Be hopeful.** Work to maintain a realistic optimism advocated by Reivich and Shatte. Misfortunes in life can lead to a broad spectrum of outcomes. The possibilities may range from mildly annoying to truly calamitous. Try to be hopeful that things will end up towards the more favorable end of what could plausibly occur. Visualize the best-case scenario rather than worrying about the worst-case scenario.

10. **Take care of yourself**. Even when you are under tremendous psychological pressure, do not neglect your basic physical and psychological needs. Eat a healthy diet and exercise regularly. Try to get some natural sunlight and spend time in nature. Be around people you love and do things you enjoy. Rest your body and mind from time to time.

CHAPTER FIVE REFERENCES

1. Rutter, M. Developing concepts in developmental psychopathology. *Developmental psychopathology and wellness: Genetic and environmental influences* 2008;pp. 3-22.
2. Lazarus RS, Folkman S. *Stress, appraisal, and coping.* New York: Springer 1984
3. Williams JMG., Watts F., MacLeod C., Mathews A. *Cognitive Psychology and Emotional Disorders.* Chichester: John Wiley & Sons, 1998
4. Diamond A. Executive Functions. *Annual Review of Psychology* 2014;64, 135–168
5. Ellis A, Harper RA. *A guide to rational living; third edition.* Melvin Powers Wilshire Book Company, 1997
6. Jovanovic T, Norrholm SD. Neural Mechanisms of Impaired Fear Inhibition in Posttraumatic Stress Disorder. *Front Behav Neurosci* 2011;5:44.
7. Friedman M, Keane T, Resick P. *Handbook of PTSD.* New York, NY: The Guilford Press, 2007
8. Brandtstädter J, Rothermund K. The Life-Course Dynamics of Goal Pursuit and Goal Adjustment: A Two-Process Framework. *Developmental Review* 2002;22(1), 117–150.
9. MacLeod C., Rutherford E., Campbell L., Ebsworthy G, Holker L. Selective attention and emotional vulnerability: Assessing the causal basis of their association through the experimental manipulation of attentional bias. *Journal of Abnormal Psychology* 2002;111(1):107–123.
10. Kubzansky L, Kiswanath K. *The Science of Happiness.* Time Magazine, 2005
11. Steptoe A, Wardle J, Marmot M. Positive affect and health-related neuroendocrine, cardiovascular, and inflam-

matory processes. *Proceedings of the National Academy of Sciences* 2005;102 (18):6508–1.

12. Danesh J, Collins R, Appleby P, Peto R. Association of fibrinogen, C-reactive protein, albumin, or leukocyte count with coronary heart disease: meta-analyses of prospective studies. *JAMA* 1998 May 13; 279(18):1477-82.

13. Frey BS. Happy People Live Longer. *Science* 2011;331 (6017): 542–43.

14. Danner DD, Snowdon DA, Friesen WV. Positive emotions in early life and longevity: Findings from the nun study. *Journal of Personality and Social Psychology* 2001;80:804–813.

15. "Positive emotions broaden the scope of attention and thought-action repertoires"; Fredrickson, B. L.; Branigan, C (2005). Cognition & Emotion. 19 (3): 313–332.

16. "On carrots and curiosity: eating fruit and vegetables is associated with greater flourishing in daily life"; Conner, Tamlin S.; Brookie, Kate L.; Richardson, Aimee C.; Polak, Maria A; British Journal of Health Psychology. 20 (2): 413–427;); 2015-05-01

17. White BA, Horwath CC, Conner TS. Many apples a day keep the blues away--daily experiences of negative and positive affect and food consumption in young adults. British *Journal of Health Psychology* 2013;18 (4): 782–798.

18. Aknin L, Norton M, Dunn E. From wealth to well-being? Money matters, but less than people think. *The Journal of Positive Psychology* 2009;4 (6): 523–7.

19. Easterlin R. Income and happiness: towards a unified theory. *The Economic Journal* 2008;11 (473): 465–484.

20. Shenk J. Finding happiness After Harvard. *Wilson Quarterly* 2009;33: 73–74.

21. Seligman MEP. *Authentic Happiness: Using the New Positive Psychology to Realize Your Potential for Lasting Fulfillment.* Free Press, 2002.

22. Hoppmann CA, Gerstorf D, Willis SL, Shaie KW. Spousal interrelations in happiness in the Seattle Longitudinal Study: Considerable similarities in levels and change over time. *Developmental Psychology* 2011;47 (1): 1–8.

23. Fowler JH, Christakis NA. Dynamic spread of happiness in a large social network: longitudinal analysis over 20 years in the Framingham Heart Study. *BMJ* 2008;337 (768): a2338

24. Loyd R. Best Benefit of Exercise? Happiness. *Fox News*, May 30, 2006.

25. Bayliss D. Physical Activity and Exercise: The Wonder Drug. *American Association of Kidney Patients*.

26. Wallis C. Science of Happiness: New Research on Mood, Satisfaction. *TIME*, February 9, 2005.

27. Twenge JM, Campbell WK, Foster CA. Parenthood and Marital Satisfaction: A Meta-Analytic Review. *Journal of Marriage and Family* 2003;65 (3): 574–583

28. Evenson RJ et al. Clarifying the Relationship Between Parenthood and Depression. Journal of Health and Social Behavior 2005;46 (4): 341–358.

29. The joys of parenthood. *The Economist,* 2008-03-27

30. Brooks AC. Gross National Happiness: Why Happiness Matters for America – and How We Can Get More of It. Basic Books, 2008.

31. Shenk J. Finding happiness After Harvard. *Wilson Quarterly* 2009;33: 73–74.

32. The science behind the smile. *Harvard business review*, 1-2, 2012

33. Seligman M. Martin Seligman: The new era of positive psychology. Ted2004; 2004

34. Archontaki D et al. Genetic influences on psychologic well being: a nationally representative Twin study. *Journal of personality* 2013;B1:2.

35. Csikszentmihalyi M. Flow: *The psychology of optimal experience*. Harper Collins, 2008.

36. Seligman M. *Flourish*. New York: Free Press, 2011;pp. 16–20.

37. Seligman MEP. Authentic Happiness: Using the new positive psychology to realize your potential for lasting fulfillment. Free Press New York; 2002

38. Frankl V. Man's Search for Meaning; An Introduction to Logotherapy. Beacon Press, Boston, MA, 2006

39. Princess Diana Quotes. BrainyQuote.com, Xplore Inc, 2017. Available at https://www.brainyquote.com/quotes/quotes/p/princessdi127197.html, accessed September 19, 2017.

40. Kobasa SC, Maddi SR, Kahn S. Hardiness and health: A prospective study. *Journal of Personality and Social Psychology* 1982;Vol 42(1):168-177

41. Maddi SR. The story of hardiness: Twenty years of theorizing, research, and practice. *Consulting Psychology Journal: Practice and Research* 2002;Vol 54(3):173-185.

42. Maddi SR. Hardiness: The courage to grow from stresses. *The journal of positive psychology*; 2006; volume 1, issue 3.

43. Schwartz CE, Sendor M. Helping others helps oneself: response shift effects in peer support. *Soc Sci Med* 1999 Jun;48(11):1563-75.

44. The Road to Resilience. *American Psychological Association*, 2014.

45. Hayes SC, Strosahl K, Wilson KG. *Acceptance and Commitment Therapy: The Process and Practice of Mindful Change*. 2nd ed New York, NY: Guilford Press; 2011.

46. Pakenham KI, Scott T, Uccelli MM. Short Report: Evaluation of Acceptance and Commitment Therapy Training for Psychologists Working with People with Multiple Sclerosis. Int J MS Care. 2018 Jan–Feb; 20(1): 44–48.

47. Pakenham KI. Training in acceptance and commitment therapy fosters self-care in clinical psychology trainees. *Clin Psychol.* 2017;21: 186– 194.

48. Richards R, Oliver JE, Morris E, Aherne K, Iervolino AC, Wingrove J. Acceptance and commitment therapy training for clinicians: an evaluation. *Cogn Behav Therapist.* 2011; 4: 114– 121.

49. Pakenham KI, Mawdsley M, Brown FL, Burton NW. Pilot evaluation of a resilience training program for people with multiple sclerosis. Rehabil Psychol 2018 Feb;63(1):29-42.

50. Harrison AM, McCracken LM, Jones K, Norton S, Moss-Morris R. Using mixed methods case-series evaluation in the development of a guided self-management hybrid CBT and ACT intervention for multiple sclerosis pain. Disabil Rehabil. 2017 Sep;39(18):1785-1798.

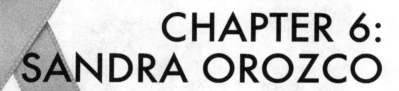

CHAPTER 6:
SANDRA OROZCO

"We will either find a way, or make one."
—Anibal Barca

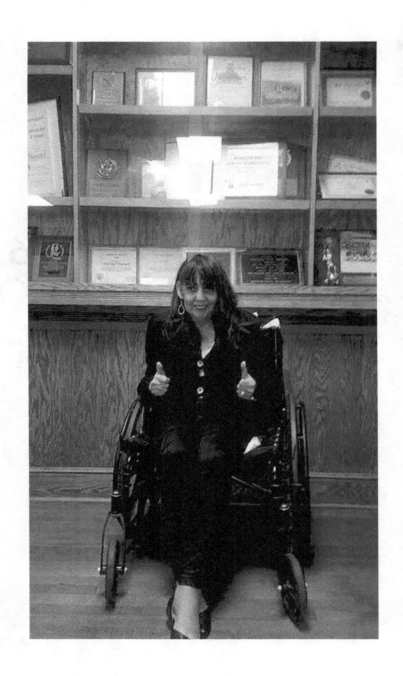

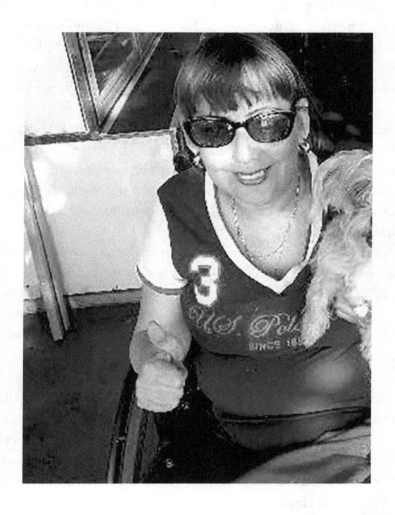

WE BRIEFLY MET Sandra Orozco at the beginning of the first Chapter. She is now a sixty-two-year-old woman with advanced progressive multiple sclerosis. She has been using a wheelchair for many years and has very limited mobility. When I picked her up for our interview, I had to manually lift her legs into my car to help her transfer from her wheelchair. However, her physical disability contrasts sharply with her dynamic personality, high energy, and incredible ambition. Long ago, she worked in health care administration, but she now spends her time as a local political activist, and she is best known for her work in voicing out against the infamous city of Bell scandal. Her story features the rise of a promising young career derailed by MS and severe depression. This setback triggered a complete restructuring of lifestyle and a reincarnation with a new life purpose.

Sandra was born at USC medical center in downtown Los Angeles in 1955. Her mother is Puerto Rican, and her father is Mexican. She is the youngest of four siblings including two older brothers and a fraternal twin sister who is a mere nineteen minutes older. Her father was born in Tucson, Arizona, but he was raised primarily in Mexico. He came back to the United States to serve in the Army, seeking opportunities his home country did not provide. While on tour in Puerto Rico, he met Sandra's mother, and they eventually married. After leaving the Army, he worked as an engineer for Douglas Aircraft, and he later owned his own small retail television business. At first, he was barely making ends meet, but he later carved out a modest living, allowing his wife to stay home and raise their four children.

My dad was a man of integrity—a hard-working man who provided for his family. He was very soft spoken; he was the shy one. My mother is Puerto Rican and has more of an aggressive personality. She's always strong and is very hard on me, so that's why we sometimes have issues, but at the end of the day, my mother cares for me. She's presently eighty-eight-years old. Sometimes, she goes astray and gets a little off track—depressed or whatever—but she has a lot of church and family support. My mom's goal was for us to do better than they did. They didn't want us going through the hardships they went through because they were very poor, but they worked hard to get the American dream which they achieved. They didn't want us to go through that, so they encouraged us to go for a career. I'm the only one that finished college, so my mother was proud of me...even proud of me today because I'm now involved in politics.

Sandra grew up in Compton, California, and she lived there until age seventeen. Compton has a deserved reputation as a rough, high-crime neighborhood, often named with pride in gangster rap lyrics. However, it now boasts an average single-family home value of over $300,000, and it probably has more cricket players than gangsters[1]. I have personally jogged after work in nearby Paramount at least a hundred times without a hint of danger. The sixties, though, were a different time, and Sandra stayed out of trouble by maintaining close ties with her family, church, and the local community. Her parents were quite religious, and many of her early memories derive from time spent in the pews of a Baptist church where much of her family's social life took place. Besides attending weekly services and joining youth groups, there were church related field trips and beach parties. She was in the choir and sang in a quartet.

One of my hobbies is to sing songs to God. That's one thing I really enjoy doing. We lived a very humble and simple life. We were always dedicated to go to church.

When Sandra was young, she was very timid and introverted, a surprising fact given her current charismatic and gregarious nature. She had selective mutism, refusing to speak in kindergarten, and she would have been placed in special education were it not for her mother's objection. Her childhood was a time of great conflict in Los Angeles. There was significant racial discrimination toward Latinos and African Americans, and she remembers the Watts riots vividly. At age seventeen, she moved to Huntington Park briefly and then to the City of Maywood, Los Angeles in 1971 where she lives today.

When she was thirteen, Sandra experienced what she believes was divine intervention that saved her life. She had been up late the night before at a prayer meeting, and she was lying in bed awake early in the morning. She lived on a major boulevard, and a car had lost control and had run through a cheap wooden fence, veering right towards her house. Unexpectedly, she felt a compulsion to get up and go into the kitchen. Then, she and her mother saw the car. They ducked their heads and heard the sounds of carnage. The car did not break through the walls, but it did significant structural damage to the outside of the house, and the impact toppled an old heavy Singer sewing machine directly onto her bed where Sandra had just been sleeping. She believes the sewing machine would have killed her were it not for God's silent message that caused her to leave her bed. This episode strengthened her faith, a force that has supported her throughout her entire life, even during her darkest moments.

In high school, Sandra focused on both academics and athletics. She swam and played baseball and volleyball. Her parents always encouraged her to work hard and act nobly, but she did not have any specific career or educational guidance because no one in her family had the experience to advise her. Despite this, everything seemed to work out. She first attended East L.A. Community College and later transferred to Cal State Los Angeles. Sandra was in love with education. She loved reading, attending lectures, and learning new things.

I was young. I was vibrant. I was fevered. I knew I had a future. My experience in college was very gratifying. I knew I was going to achieve my goals, and I did reach the goals, until I was hit with multiple sclerosis. Multiple sclerosis changed my life forever, even as we speak.

She studied voraciously but still had time to make many new friends and to compete on an amateur gymnastics team. She ended up getting into the field of health care administration, an important and rapidly growing field with increasing opportunities due to the growing complexity of health care billing and regulation. Having a passion for things most find mundane and bureaucratic, she loved health care and the language of medicine. She is a natural leader—energetic, organized, and able to appreciate how the system benefits the individual.

Sandra was obsessed with work. She would attend meetings and set up workshops to educate the novices entering the field. This hardly left time for a personal life, and much of her socializing connected with church and her workplace. To advance in medical management, she had to give up many of the hobbies of her youth, and her love life was always on the back burner.

I can't have a man. I just can't. I'm too busy. To have a man in your life is to have another job because you have to work on that relationship. I have a relationship with Jesus, so I don't need a man; I'm married to him. So, I find myself setting out to help people, and that's what's important. I came to this world to help people.

Despite this sentiment, she eventually did find time for a little romance. She met a man named Daniel at a social gathering related to her work. He was an attorney representing a major hospital, and Sandra was working on legal issues related to medical records. They were immediately drawn to each other, and she was particularly attracted to his dynamic personality and big blue eyes. He was congenial, dependable, and well-heeled. He owned a boat, and they used to take trips to Catalina. He seemed like the perfect man, and she seriously contemplated marrying him. They were together for two years before it all came crashing down when she found out he was seeing someone else.

He was a good man, but he cheated on me. When somebody cheats on me, they're not welcome in my world. It's better that he cheated on me then, because I believe in marriage. I believe in "'til death do us part." If I marry somebody, it's for life—because that's what the Bible says it should be. Not only that, but I have the example of my parents.

She had other dates and boyfriends, but nothing ever materialized into a significant relationship. Her work, friends, family, and church dominated her attention. She has a large family and a larger community, and she never had difficulty filling her schedule.

In her late twenties, Sandra was the victim of a drive-by shooting. She was on the freeway when she heard a barrage of gunshots which echoed within her vehicle. Because of the shock of the incident, she lost control of her car and spun. She later pulled over and found a few bullet-holes in the side of her car and a few casings that flew through her window. Luckily, she was completely uninjured. California highway patrol came to question her, but they never resolved the case. To this day, she does not know if she survived an attempted murder or if she was a random recipient of misfire. She considers herself lucky and sees the event as confirmation that God is watching over her. However, she would later learn that even the faithful can face the mightiest of challenges.

Sandra developed her first symptoms of MS when she was thirty-eight years old. It was January 19th, 1993. It happened so long ago she cannot recall the exact sequence of events, but she retains a vivid memory of what it felt like to be overtaken by the mysterious illness. Her symptoms were vague at first, and she noticed a slight sense of imbalance. Soon after, she developed vertigo and had un-explained episodes of passing out. Then, her condition deteriorated rapidly, and she had a series of relapses back to back. She had an unusual diffuse pain which in retrospect we recognize was neuro-pathic pain.

My head was spinning. I was in severe pain. On a scale of one to ten, it was a twenty. I couldn't even turn my head to the left because I was in such pain. I had paralysis of my right face. My throat had closed down, and I could not eat. I had peripheral blindness of both eyes. I felt like I was dying. I lost faith. I lost hope. I lost my career as a healthcare profes-sional. I was slowly going into a state of depression, and I felt worthless to society.

She saw various doctors, and at first, the diagnosis was unclear. The uncertainty and fear were as devastating as the illness itself as she had no explanation and no path to recovery. She eventually had MRI scans and a spinal tap which revealed findings highly typical of MS. They finally gave her an answer, but the blow of the diag-nosis was crushing. She was living such a fast-paced and productive life that MS seemed to take everything away from her. At first, she found it impossible to adapt. Her initial relapses were very severe, and it would be a full year before she could even drive a car again. Around June 1993, she slowly started to recover. Her ability to swallow food normalized, and she began to regain the weight she had lost.

In the meantime, life seemed to pass her by. She was spending much of her time at home, wallowing in despair and wondering why MS had happened to her. Her ambitions and dreams were fading while her friends and siblings were thriving. Sandra's sister became an accomplished professional pianist. One of her brothers is a manager for ADT (a home security company), and her oth-er brother is a professional guitarist for a church. Sandra was near rock-bottom in terms of depression when her sister gave birth to Jonathan, her nephew. Her interaction with him gives a sense of how ill and hopeless she felt.

I went to Jonathan when he was seven days old, and I said to him, "I'm not going to be around. I'm going to be a little angel watching over you."

Sandra recounts with pleasure that she lived to form a relationship with her nephew and to see him graduate from college. He will always have a special place in her heart because of the circumstances of their first meeting. This meeting proved to be a turning point in both her physical and mental health. Ultimately, Sandra's pessimism faded when her condition began to improve. Her parents supported her through the whole process, and they encouraged her to go back to work.

Her hospital contract had expired, and she switched gears and got a job as a sub-contractor with the Ranchos Los Amigos healthcare system. She worked at Centinela Hospital and other institutions as a senior internal auditor, helping the hospitals comply with government and insurance regulations. While there, she was responsible for peer review and for keeping surveyors happy. She would attend meetings, prepare statistical reports, and perform audits. She became an expert in HIPPA compliance and "do not use" abbreviations. Her team was responsible for quality of care analysis, looking at immunizations, mammograms, and certain disease-specific interventions. Again, her career was flourishing. Even though she was not physically one-hundred percent, she had no major functional limitations. Through hard work, she gradually built a solid reputation and started receiving larger assignments. She obtained more specialized training and went out to other hospitals for investigations and teaching. She was traveling frequently, making good money, and gaining valuable experience.

Unfortunately, her contract with Ranchos Los Amigos expired in 1996, and she was no longer needed in her current role. So, the position was closed, and she lost her job. Her MS symptoms were also worsening around this time, but the depression and malaise were worse than the disease. She had low energy, lack of interest in hobbies and friends, and other typical symptoms of neurovegetative depression. Even her family seemed to give up on her, and she recounts some conversations she had with her mother at the time.

"You're fat. You're ugly. Your teeth are bad...no man's gonna want you. You're no good for nobody." My mom said that. It was verbal abuse. She plays favorites. She sides with her oldest son, so you couldn't talk about William. If I would say something, she would hit me. Even to this day, my mom says, "You should have a house. You should have a man." Well, when you are in that environment, you don't know you have that syndrome. I was crying. I would not take a bath. I didn't care about myself or my acquaintances. I didn't want to go out. I didn't want to eat.

Sandra became paranoid and emotionally unstable, irrationally afraid of the police coming to arrest her when cars would pass by. At one point, she broke down, and the police were called. They took her to a psychiatric hospital on a 5150, a seventy-two-hour involuntary admission.

Sandra remembers being interviewed by interns, psychologists, and psychiatrists. They started various medications and performed extensive counseling. It was an intimidating environment, but she felt the overwhelming support of her family. As soon as they admitted her, everyone came to visit. Even her ex-boyfriend Daniel came to see her, but she turned him away with impunity. Her mother demanded she be released even though she was the person who originally called the police. Ultimately, it was her twin sister who convinced the doctors to release her after a six-day inpatient admission. Like so many victims of depression before her, Sandra had touched the depths of hell, but she managed to land on her feet.

She then returned to work as a subcontractor in health care administration. She again worked at Centinela Hospital, and she also had projects within Kaiser facilities. Her battles with depression continued over the next decade, but she never again saw the inside of an inpatient ward. In 2000, her father died of prostate cancer and complications of chronic obstructive pulmonary disease. She lost a voice of calm encouragement and one of her primary role models during a very difficult time. Her mother was also devastated, and she never remarried. Sandra did not truly remit from depression until 2006, but she kept it under control and moved on with her life.

Her MS was stable for a period, but in the late 1990s and early 2000s, she began to slowly decline. With progressive MS, the changes are often so insidious that we only recognize them retrospectively, and Sandra followed this pattern. At first, she had trouble walking long distances and was slightly clumsy. In the mid-2000s, she began to require assistance with a cane. By 2008, she could still walk and drive, but she needed a walker. In 2011, she started using a wheelchair. At first, it was only for use over longer distances, but her disability evolved, and the wheelchair became a constant requirement. By the time I met her in 2016, she could hardly hold herself up and could only take a few awkward steps with a walker. She requires too much assistance to make walking practical on a routine basis, so for all intents and purposes, she uses a wheelchair full time. Images of Sandra's MRI scans from early 2017 are below:

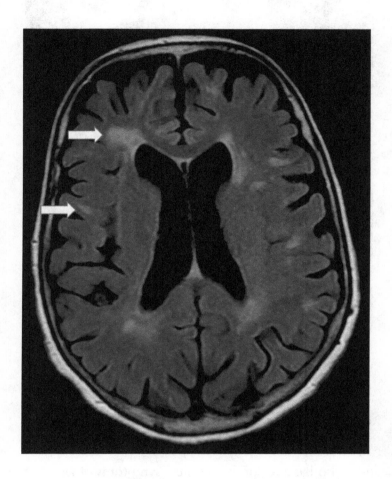

Figure 1: A T2 axial FLAIR image from an MRI of the brain revealing typical multiple sclerosis plaques. A few plaques are marked by arrows.

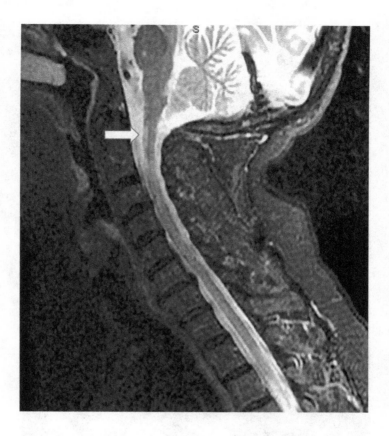

Figure 2: A T2 sagittal STIR MRI of the cervical spine revealing scattered cord lesions and cord atrophy. One lesion is marked by an arrow.

Sandra also has a lot of the invisible symptoms of MS. Although you would not know it by her rapid speech and imposing confidence, she suffers from very significant fatigue. Exhaustion builds during the day and forces her to take naps most afternoons. When exposed to the heat, she deteriorates quickly, both mentally and physically. Her legs are stiff and often cramp. Luckily, the severe neuropathic pain which plagued her in the 1990s never returned.

She was untreated during much of the course of her illness, mostly by her own choice. During the 1990s and early 2000s, she had only spotty treatment with disease modifying therapy, and many of the details are lost from her memory. The year they diagnosed her with MS, 1993, was coincidentally the year that the first disease modifying therapy for MS became FDA approved. Betaseron© was scarce and expensive, so patients had to enter a lottery to get the drug[2]. It caused side-effects and was not particularly effective, so either by choice or by lack of success in the lottery, most patients in the first few years went without treatment.

In 2008, Sandra started Avonex©, but it did not seem to alter her slow decline. She switched to Copaxone© in 2010 which she continued on until about 2014. At this point, she gave up on the shots as they seemed futile. The failure of the injections to prevent the worsening weakness in her legs was unquestionable. An MS specialist at Ranchos Los Amigos encouraged her to continue treatment, but she refused because the drugs did not seem to make much of a difference.

Sandra is not apathetic or naturalistic, but she is not much of a self-advocate when it comes to her own health. I had great trouble trying to get her to complete updated MRI scans, and she was reluctant to make the effort to obtain outside records. She seems to care more about her work and helping others than about taking care of herself. I do not mean to imply she would be less physically disabled had she received different medical treatment. This is impossible to know, and many with MS have experienced a similar course even with continuous immunotherapy[3-5]. In the last few years, she has been relatively stable despite the lack of help from modern medicine.

Sandra was able to continue working in health care for a long period, but by 2008, her mobility had worsened to where she could no longer perform her duties. Her employer had been understanding and accommodating, but she had no choice except to go out on disability. This time, her transition away from working life was not as emotionally taxing. Her disability had evolved gradually, and this tends to make the pill easier to swallow. She became accustomed to her problems and was mentally stronger than she used to be. Her experience of fifteen years with MS taught her how to be resilient, and she knew she had to find a way to stay active and productive. Her transition into political activism started when a good friend of hers invited her to a Maywood city council meeting.

City council meetings are usually mundane affairs, and discussions often involve trivialities like street sign colors and parking policies. However, Sandra continued to attend, and she gradually learned the people and the system. She befriended Jack Edels, a city of Cudahy councilmember. She worked with Valentino Mesquizo, an official from Huntington Park. She also worked with Leticia Vasquez, the municipal water director of the central basin. Everyone of political significance in Maywood and its neighboring cities seems to know her. The names and connections flow on and on. She is distinctly vibrant and charismatic, so she quickly became popular and respected in this new arena. Before 2008, she cared about politics, but she knew nothing about the intricacies of local political affairs. She began researching contemporary issues, trying to become an expert on everything and everyone.

I love education. I still do. Knowledge is power. I look to the internet to get facts. I absolutely have to get facts to prove things that are right. That's why I'm very credible. I have good morals and ethics, and that's why I do what I do. I can't be bought by politicians. I'm not a paid political activist.

Her local influence blossomed when Al Hutchings became the interim chief of the Maywood Police Department in 2008. Sandra and several others recoiled when they found out Hutchings was previously convicted of theft and had resigned from the Los Angeles Police department. He also had been fired from Los Angeles Valley College in 2005, reportedly for acts of dishonesty[6]. Sandra spoke out aggressively against the appointment of Hutchings at council meetings. Within a few weeks, the mayor of Maywood asked the interim chief to step down, and a new interim chief replaced him[7]. The media interviewed Sandra about the incident, and it brought a lot of attention to corruption within the Maywood Police force.

However, Sandra did not truly become known within the local southeast political community until the City of Bell Scandal. This occurred in 2010, enraging the community and turning into a national news story. The city manager, Robert Rizzo, and the assistant chief administrative officer, Angela Spaccia, were abusing their power to pay themselves outrageous salaries from the city's scarce funds. Robert Rizzo himself collected over $1,000,000 per year[8], an absurd salary for a manager of a tiny city with only 35,000 people.

The entire city council was in on the scheme, and they went to great lengths to cover their tracks[8-11]. However, Sandra knew there was a problem because she found out the nearby City of Maywood had gone bankrupt and could not afford their city insurance. She became suspicious that the problem could relate to Angela Spaccia who had become acting city manager for Maywood. Sandra then tipped off Ruben Vives, a friend and journalist of the LA times. Vives investigated further and broke the story in a series of damning articles.

Bell residents erupted with protest, and Sandra was on the front lines, speaking publicly and gathering support. She remembers confronting the perpetrators at a televised city council meeting shortly before their arrests.

I'll never forget the day that I went up there. I was in my walker, and I go up to the podium. There were tons of people. The media was there. "You're a damned liar! You need to go to jail, and you need to go to jail right now!" And so I prophesied. Within ten hours, that's what the FBI did: they took all of them.

At the end of the day, the evidence from personal e-mails was overwhelming, and the defendants were crushed at trial. Rizzo, Spaccia, and several members from the city council spent years in prison[12-15]. After the dust settled, Sandra Orozco became well known within Maywood politics, and the entire city had a renewed political fervor. For a more detailed account of the Bell scandal, see **appendix B.**

For the most part, justice was served, but Sandra still suspects a connection between the Bell scandal and Maywood's financial woes. Her beloved city still suffers from the aftermath of chronic mismanagement, and she believes several others rightfully belong in jail. From this incident, she has developed a passion for good government and accountability, and she considers herself a watchdog over corrupt businesses and politicians. The unscrupulousness in the southeast has unfortunately continued. In 2013, David Silva, the former mayor of Cudahy, was sentenced to federal prison for accepting bribes from a marijuana dispensary[16]. David and Sandra were friends, so the news blindsided her.

I used to talk to him. Seek God, David. Seek God. For some reason, he didn't do what I told him to do, and he ends up getting wired by the FBI. What happened, David? I would have given you the five thousand.

Sandra has supported various political projects over the years. She continues to attend council meetings at Maywood along with meetings at nearby Bell, Cudahy, and Huntington Park. She also attends school board meetings at Los Angeles Unified. Her schedule is amazingly busy for a disabled person, filled with meetings, dinners, phone conversations, and researching on the internet. She has become familiar not just with the individual issues but with the language, bureaucracy, and personnel of local southeast politics.

She has investigated Maywood Mutual Water Company No. 1 and 2 and advocated for a unified district manager. She helped to encourage the development of a surgery center in Huntington Park and is trying to get funding for a new hospital to replace the aging Huntington Park Community Hospital. She is urging for a police substation in the City of Maywood to make up for the lost local police department. In 2014, Sandra warned the Huntington Park city council about lead and arsenic emissions from the Exide Battery Recycling Factory[17], and there is significant evidence for the connection between Exide and increased soil lead levels and arsenic emissions[18]. There were various local reports of elevated lead levels in children with developmental delays. In March 2015, the Exide plant shut down in a deal with the justice department, and they forced the company to pay $50,000,000 in restitution[18].

In 2015, she spoke out against the illegal hiring of two undocumented immigrants as commissioners on city advisory boards in Huntington Park[19]. The council stood accused of handing out open contracts to friends and hiring relatives to advisory committees. Sandra and her cohort attended council meetings to hold up signs and demand resignations. In February 2016, she and other dissatisfied residents served recall papers to four Huntington Park council members[20].

> It's what you call "play by pay." This is like déjà vu. This is unreal. They have a city manager currently. He's no good. He has no experience. He's getting paid over $200,000. You don't think the FBI is looking at you guys? Oh yeah...you'll be the next ones in the news. Your asses are gonna be in jail.

Sandra also has concerns about the school system in Maywood and Bell. Because of current overcrowding, the students work an unusual year-round schedule[21]. Sandra and her contemporaries have been pushing for new construction for many years. In February 2015, the City broke ground on a new South Region High School which they completed in 2017[22]. Sandra hopes the students will return to a regular track system, allowing them to have summers off and discouraging them from dropping out.

Sandra did not initiate many of these projects, but she is a great builder of political momentum and helps to connect the desires of the people to local politicians. She is the most vocal member of a small group of like-minded activists, and they use various tactics to achieve their political objectives. Much of their influence is by word of mouth through extensive social networks. They send fliers to registered voters, cause a stir at council meetings, protest in large groups with vivid signs, and give sound bites to the media. She has forged relationships with local media members such as CBS reporter Dave Bryan, and she communicates with them via text message regularly. She also has connections with NBC, Telemundo, Univision, ABC, Fox, The Los Angeles Times, La Voz, La Opinión, The Wave Newspaper, EstrellaTV, and KTLA. In 2016, the Los Angeles County Democratic Party voted Sandra one of the Roosevelt Democrats of the year[23]. Many of her friends have encouraged her to pursue a leadership position herself, and she is thinking about running for the Mayor of Maywood.

Even at sixty-one, she does not have much of her life planned out. She may run for mayor, though this is only a fantasy for the time being. She was also considering applying to law school and getting into the legal side of politics. At some point, she wants to write an autobiography about her life and her struggle with MS. She has considered becoming a motivational speaker as well. Her living situation is just as unsettled as her professional aspirations. She previously lived in her mother's home, but given the tensions between them, she is currently living alone in a nearby apartment. She dreams of owning her own home in the city of Maywood which she hopes to achieve within the next few years.

Although she keeps a busy schedule, she tries to make time for her personal interests and hobbies. Sandra seems to have a thousand friends and acquaintances, and while I was with her in Maywood,

I got the sense she knew everyone and was known by everyone in the city. She likes talking to random people in the community and learning about their lives. It is routine for her to meet strangers and to pray for them. She sings, plays piano by ear, and reads scripture. Even with her physical limitations, she can still swim regularly as her main form of exercise. She loves jazz music and other forms of entertainment, and she likes to visit the zoo and the beach. She is a hopeless foodie, and our interview took place at an authentic Mexican restaurant, causing me to break my normally strict diet.

One amazing thing about Sandra is she is completely self-sufficient. She pays her own bills and takes care of her own hygiene, shopping, housework, and transportation. Well-networked and street smart, she is not afraid to ask a friend for a ride or a favor. Subsidized transportation programs like Access and Cudahy Dollar Ride help as well. A few simple adaptations like a special railing to lift herself out of bed allow her to live on her own. To put on her shoes, she must reach down to lift her legs. She goes to local markets frequently, carrying back what she can in a single trip. Family, personal friends, political friends, and church friends help her when she faces a roadblock trying to complete a simple errand we all take for granted. Her disability is sufficiently longstanding that these things have become routine and trivial, barely worthy of mention. She looks at the big picture, not the little details. Perhaps this is to a fault as she is so busy with local politics that she lacks a certain long-term organization and linearity in her life plans. However, she just focuses on the present, and everything seems to work out for her. She also does not think much about what her life would have been like without MS. She shows no particular concern with money, her long lost career, romance, and the other typical aspirations associated with a "normal" life.

I don't need all of those materialistic things. I'm happy with what I am. I have joy. I have kindness. I have self-control. I have peace. I have love.

I have compassion. I'm in a wheelchair, and I have my challenges with MS, but MS can't stop me. Multiple sclerosis can't stop this Maywood activist. I never get mad...knowing that there are people being diagnosed with cancer, and they're dying as we speak. There are children that are dying. There are people in third world countries that don't have water or food.

As expected for anyone in her condition, Sandra has gone through tough times, but she has held off her previously crippling depression for the last eleven years. When she needs inspiration, she looks to the memory of her father and to local political leaders she admires like Pat Acosta and Leticia Vasquez. Most of all, she looks to her faith in God.

My faith in God has been with me since I was a child. I am who I am today because the Bible says, "Seek ye first the kingdom of God and its righteousness and all these things shall be on to you" and "What's impossible with man is possible with God." So, I key into verses on the providence of God, and that's what motivates me to keep going on and on. I trust in God's promises. God tells us to have joy in salvation and that He gives us peace. That's what gives me joy. That's what brings me happiness and brings me calm. When I fail, I say, "Forgive me God," and I pick up the pieces so I can go forward. God is my resource; He's my helper. He's the person I depend on. He's the song in my morning and at night. I pray to Him even during my challenges in life. I can do all things through Christ who strengthens me, and I have a praying mother that prays for me all the time. I continually put faith in God, and I know God is there.

Besides her faith in God, Sandra has many of the characteristics of resilience discussed in Chapter Three. Although she speaks with a fire-bellied fervor at political rallies, she is mostly in control of her emotions. She is calm, patient, and analytical when she needs to be. When she feels herself becoming upset or angry, she mentally counts to ten and takes a deep breath. She is also a deeply optimistic person. Despite everything that has happened to her and all the negative news in the local political arena, she views her own future as bright and genuinely believes the local southeast community is on the economic and sociopolitical rise. She knows there will always be crooks and incompetents, but there are also amazingly talented and industrious politicians whom she admires and commends.

Sandra believes in causal analysis, and she has confidence in her ability to make a meaningful change. She spends much of her time pilfering through news articles and researching issues, and she believes if she can understand the root cause of problems, she is well on the way to solving them. Because of all she has gone through with both her illness and her family, she is naturally empathetic to others—those that are disenfranchised, victimized, sick, and tired. She has a unique sensitivity to the poor, the broken-hearted, and the abused because she herself is a survivor. She also has a great ability to build a community around her. Although she is an independent spirit, she is humble and quick to seek local support. She has achieved a paragon of what Stephen Covey would call "interdependence."

She also has filled her life with the engagement and meaning advocated by Dr. Seligman. So busy with the present, she hardly has time to think about the past or future. She is constantly traveling around town, meeting new people, and reading about politics, so she rarely thinks about the inconveniences of MS. Just as I unintentionally skip lunch when I am busy in my clinic, she unintentionally skips self-pity when busy with life. Thus, she has crafted a deeply meaningful life with a continuous sense of purpose. Part of this comes from her religious conviction, and another part comes from her involvement in politics. Overcoming her immobility and fatigue is hard, but she always has a reason to rise above. There is always a voice in the back of her head saying, "Keep moving, Sandra. What you are doing is important. The world needs you."

Sandra's story teaches us that resilience is not merely an innate and stagnant characteristic. If I had met her in her forties at the nadir of depression, I would have seen her in an entirely different light. At the time, she was only marginally disabled and had plenty of opportunity, but the MS and depression were crushing. Somehow, her humble background, Christian work ethic, and strong social support system were not enough for her. However, these are the exact factors to which she credits her resilience later in life. She had to suffer through the hard times, reinvent herself, and forge resilience over years and decades. She simply did not have this type of experience early in life, and when MS first hit her, it was so vicious and unearthing that she did not know how to deal with it. She teaches us that resilience is a complex phenomenon related to one's personality, experiences, and specific latitude in life.

Just like Dr. Spitz, she had a hard-working and encouraging father. Just like Dr. Bhat, she had conservative parents with strong values and specific expectations of her. However, the two doctors only had subtle symptoms at the time of diagnosis, and this made the diagnosis of MS much easier to accept. Neither of them had to face a seemingly catastrophic onset of symptoms. Sandra fared much when her MS was progressive because she had time to adapt to the changes.

Also, I think there is a similarity between Sandra and James Bhat: they both tend to downplay and disregard their symptoms. They both have an unusual form of utilitarian apathy. This is essentially the same as the accommodative coping response I discussed in the previous chapter. There are disadvantages to this, of course. Sandra did not have a medical background, a supportive spouse, or an enfranchised family to help her get medical care, so she was untreated for much of her illness. She likely would have recovered more rapidly from her first attack with a prompt diagnosis and intravenous steroids, and this might have stopped her spiral into depression. She did not even consider using the newer drugs when they came onto the market. In fact, she has not even heard of most of them. Nor did she receive physical therapy during much of her tenure with the disease. When I met her for the first time in my office, she was more interested in talking about her personal life than about MS. She was not looking for a cure or even for a way to ameliorate her most meddlesome symptoms. She does not research MS or go to MS support groups. As a result, she is not very knowledgeable about the disease considering her intelligence, level of education, and longevity with the illness.

However, all of this may be to her advantage because it allows her to focus on other aspects of her existence. She chooses to battle life rather than MS, and this prevents her from becoming overwhelmed by the disease. Even though she is an advocate for people with MS, she does not want to be known for her MS. She wants to be known as a good Christian, a loyal friend, and a southeast political activist. She has certainly convinced me, and I am just one of thousands of people who were lucky enough to cross her path in life and learn from her experiences. Sandra inspired me to become interested in local politics, and she changes the way I think about the meaning of my life. When I am having a rough day, I try to think about her vibrant spirit, genuine virtue, and infectious smile. Undoubtedly, we could all use a little Sandra Orozco within us.

CHAPTER 6 REFERENCES

1. Takahashi C. The Compton You Haven't Seen On Screen. *NPR*, August 13, 2015. Available at http://www.npr.org/2015/08/13/431907210/the-compton-you-havent-seen-on-screen.

2. Lewin T. Experimental Drug Is Prize In a Highly Unusual Lottery. *The New York Times*, January 7, 1994

3. La Mantia L, Munari LM, Lovati R. Glatiramer acetate for multiple sclerosis. *Cochrane Database Syst Rev* 2010, Issue 5.

4. La Mantia L, Vacchi L, Di Pietrantonj C, Ebers G, Rovaris M, Fredrikson S, Filippini G. Interferon beta for secondary progressive multiple sclerosis. *Cochrane Database Syst Rev* 2012, Issue 1.

5. Rojas JI, Romano M, Ciapponi A, Patrucco L, Cristiano E. Interferon Beta for Primary Progressive Multiple Sclerosis. *Cochrane Database Syst Rev* 2010, Issue 1

6. Lait M, Convicted cop hired as police chief; Maywood hires the ex-LAPD officer over opposition from the rank and file and the city's attorney. *LA Times*, February 02, 2008.

7. Bloomekatz AB. Controversial chief in Maywood steps down. *LA Times*, February 13, 2008

8. 214 Cal.App.4th 921; Court of Appeal, Second District, Division 3, California. The PEOPLE EX REL. Kamala D. HARRIS, as Attorney General, etc., Plaintiff and Appellant, v. Robert A. RIZZO et al., Defendants and Respondents.; B236246; Filed March 20, 2013

9. 209 Cal.App.4th 93; Court of Appeal, Second District, Division 3, California.; Pier'Angela SPACCIA, Petitioner, v. The SUPERIOR COURT of Los Angeles County, Respondent, People of the State of California, Real Parties in

Interest. No. B239472.; Sept. 6, 2012.; As Modified Sept. 25, 2012.

10. Gov.Code, § 36516, subd. (a)(2)(B).

11. Vives R, Gottlieb J. Is a city manager worth $800,000? *LA Times*, July, 15 2010

12. Knoll C, Mather K. Former Bell official Angela Spaccia gets 11 years, 8 months in prison. *LA Times*, April 10, 2014.

13. Jahad S. Sentenced to 12 years in state prison, $9 million in restitution. *KPCC with Associated Press*, April 16 2014.

14. Los Angeles Times Staff. Bell Corruption verdicts. *LA Times*; March 20, 2013.

15. Knoll C. Former Bell Councilwoman Teresa Jacobo gets two-year prison sentence. *LA Times*, July 25, 2014.

16. Gottlieb J. Ex-Cudahy mayor gets prison in bribes. *LA Times*, January 29, 2013.

17. Chibarirwe A. Huntington Park and the Slippery Slope of Illegal Immigration. *The new legal*, August 6, 2015.

18. Barboza T. Higher levels of lead found in blood of children near Exide plant in Vernon. *LA Times*, April 8, 2016

19. City Council Agenda Monday, January 6, 2014. City of Huntington Park. Available at http://www.hpca.gov/ArchiveCenter/ViewFile/Item/2967

20. Adler A. Recall notices served on Huntington Park council members. *Wave Newspapers*, February 19, 2016

21. Watanabe T. These LAUSD students are not heading back to school. *LA Times*, August 17, 2015.

22. Wave staff. Construction to begin on Maywood school. *Los Angeles Wave*, January 31, 2015

23. 2016 Roosevelt Democrats of the year. Available at http://www.lacdp.org/honorees/

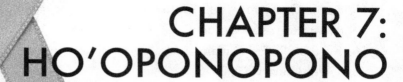

CHAPTER 7:
HO'OPONOPONO

*"Many times happiness is just around the corner,
on that corner that we never dare to turn."*
— Mabel Katz, *The Easiest Way Special Edition*

SOMETIMES IN MEDICINE, we focus so much on disease and complicated treatment regimens that we neglect the patient's general health and mental state. If the medical encounter is too encumbered with discussions of diagnosis, examination, and pharmaceuticals, what time is there to discuss resilience? What time is there for the intangible human component of disease? According to some osteopathic practitioners, even the "term, 'patient,' and the manner in which we gather biopsychosocial data, for example, implies a reduction of the person to a passive recipient of health-care"[1]. For a trauma patient requiring emergency surgery, a passive approach works just fine, but for chronic conditions like MS, active participation can make all the difference in the world. Resilience in the face of illness is something which we should foster in the medical setting, but we often lack the desire, training, and resources to do this.

Perhaps developing resilience is something that comes more from the wisdom and experience of human culture over generations than from modern scientific research. One traditional philosophy that deals with the attitude towards conflict in life is the Polynesian practice of Ho'oponopono. I came across Ho'oponopono by chance, and I had never even heard of it before I started writing this book. When I read about it more deeply, I realized it brings a new perspective to the concept of resilience. The modern practice of Ho'oponopono is a method of "self-identity" and approaching the world in a new way. It is practiced mostly in the US (especially Hawaii), Europe, Asia, Dubai, and Australia[2]. The term Ho'oponopono literally means "to make right, orderly, and correct"[3], and it is a process of forgiveness, appreciation, and refocusing. The ideology asks practitioners to give thanks, give love, and to ask for forgiveness.

Ho'oponopono encourages you to take responsibility for everything in life including your attitude towards the world and how you treat people. You should accept conflict as an opportunity to improve yourself and to change your life. Proponents believe subconscious thoughts and automated responses drive people toward negative attitudes and patterns of behavior. Because of this, you must clear your mind of negative thoughts and replace them with love, requests for forgiveness, and gratitude. While Ho'oponopono is a general life philosophy, it has been used specifically to solve family conflicts. In scientific studies, it has been found to lower blood pressure[2] and to help with the psychological adaptation to breast cancer.

The idea of self-responsibility is a powerful thing. I remember a time when I was a first-year medical student, and I saw a patient who was very obese with severe arthritis of the knees. My preceptor told her plainly and bluntly, "You will not get better unless you lose one-hundred pounds!" The patient immediately asked if we could admit her to the hospital in a controlled weight loss program. Of course, my preceptor informed her he could not do this, and he proceeded to give her dietary advice. I asked him afterwards if he thought she would succeed, and he told me, "Of course not; she's looking for the easy way out." At the time, I thought he was cold and cynical, but after having had hundreds of conversations with patients about weight loss, I have learned that my old mentor was right. People rarely succeed in losing weight unless they genuinely and whole-heartedly believe they are responsible for their fate and have the power to change. You must look in the mirror and say, "I can do it; my actions will determine the outcome. No one else and no external force will stop me from achieving my goals." This does not mean one cannot seek outside help or look for the most efficient route, but you simply cannot skip the first step of self-accountability.

Self-responsibility and accountability is a useful paradigm in almost any aspect of life. When is it better to believe the world is conspiring against you or that the whims of others and your arbitrary circumstances are more important than your personal decisions?

Surely, I must concede that no one is in complete control of her circumstances. This is more evident now than it ever has been in human history. We are subject to the consequences of the actions of so many people around us whom we cannot control. Our lot in life is influenced by the country we are born in, the resources of our family, our early education, our coworkers, our friends, our bosses, and perhaps most of all, our health. We are much more aware of this than an early American settler building a log cabin with his bare hands. How can one think about self-responsibility after being diagnosed with a seemingly random and poorly understood disease? This is the very reason we go astray.

The point about self-responsibility is more about pragmatism than reality. Self-responsibility is useful on a day-to-day basis. Let us assume, for the sake of argument, that the obese woman with arthritis has both a slow metabolism and a poor diet. Which one would be more useful to think about? Should she wallow in despair over being cursed with a poor metabolism or should she take responsibility for her dietary choices? The former appeals to the ego, but the latter is more actionable. The author Mabel Katz calls this idea "one-hundred percent responsibility" and argues that this is actually "the easiest way" to approach life[4]. Having one-hundred percent responsibility is having complete freedom and having confidence you cannot be stopped by fear, competition, or your own limitations. Although you may feel that you have limited control over your life, this has more to do with subjective perception than objective reality. Is your boss dissatisfied because of her unreasonable expectations or are your poor communication skills at fault? Is your spouse uncompromising, or is it you who is too rigid? When we experience these conflicts in real time, it seems so obvious others are at fault, but this bias is the nature of the human condition. Things are much more subjective than they seem. Remember, even a man forced into the gas chamber chooses his final thoughts before his death. It is all a matter of how you think about it, and having one-hundred percent responsibility is a very powerful thing. You will naturally become more introspective and less critical of others if you develop this mindset.

However, the purpose of Ho'oponopono is not self-condemnation, so you must ask yourself for forgiveness. One mantra of Ho'oponopono is, "I'm sorry. Please forgive me. Thank you. I love you"[5]. We say this to ourselves or to others. One proponent of Ho'oponopono, Dr. Joe Vitale, believes part of the philosophy is to achieve "the state of zero," becoming devoid of memory and identity to extrude guilt, negative thought patterns, and negative experiences. This derives from the traditional idea of karma and can be a meditative process. He believes underlying subconscious fears and insecurities can sabotage one's conscious intentions and beliefs.

Another principle of Ho'oponopono is that of giving thanks. You should show appreciation towards yourself, to others, and to God. Be thankful for your own abilities and circumstances even if things have not gone well recently. Show respect for the kind acts and talents of those around you. Although it sounds somewhat sappy, gratitude has profound internal and external benefits. If you focus on the good things in your life and the good aspects of yourself, the tough times will become more bearable. You must convince yourself everything is a blessing in disguise. Being grateful and appreciative of others naturally draws people towards you and helps you to form friendships and alliances. It is important to let people know about their admirable traits and good deeds. Take the advice of Dale Carnegie, the author of *How to Win Friends and Influence People*:

Be hearty in your approbation and lavish in your praise.[6]

Giving thanks is what Lou Gehrig did when he delivered his famous farewell address after being diagnosed with the disease that bears his name:

Fans, for the past two weeks, you have been reading about the bad break I got. Yet today, I consider myself the luckiest man on the face of this earth. I have been in ballparks for seventeen years and have never received anything but kindness and encouragement from you fans.[7]

Imagine the mindset Mr. Gehrig had in making this statement. He chose to focus on the positives in his life rather than his progressive and incurable disease. Imagine also how the crowd must have reacted to his statement. Envision a random fan who was daydreaming about the troubles in his marriage, family, or small business. Think about how trivial this all must have seemed compared to facing Lou Gehrig's disease. We have all learned Lou Gehrig's lesson many times, but it is somehow impossible to retain. We need to remind ourselves over and over again.

I remember a time when I was hospitalized with pneumonia. I did the typical thing that doctors do: keep working with shaking chills and a fever of 103.5°F and end up getting admitted straight to the intensive care unit. I got worse and worse, and I was so uncomfortable and short of breath that I genuinely feared death. However, on the third day of hospitalization, I turned the corner and slowly recovered. I had been training for a marathon before the illness derailed my plans, and I was eager to get back in to shape. I started my own rehabilitation while I was still in the hospital as soon as I was healthy enough to do so by taking walks around the hallway. After discharge, I would walk up and down the steps in my apartment building. Later, I took walks in the neighborhood with a few brief interspersed jogs. Finally, I remember the very first day when I could run. It was a snail's pace and only a few miles, but the Los Angeles air smelled like Alaska, and the runner's high was amazing. I had a newfound appreciation for running comparable to when I took up the sport at age sixteen. However, this feeling only lasted a month before I started to take it for granted.

My failure is a common one. Memory fades, and we become accustomed to our surroundings. Our lifestyle seems "normal," and anything less desirable becomes unacceptable. If I randomly teleported a typical American into a middle-class lifestyle in 15th century Europe, they would have great difficulty adjusting to it, even accounting for culture-shock. Illness can have a similar effect, and that is why it can be so devastating psychologically. No one plans on becoming ill. We imagine that everything will work out perfectly. As I write this, I can so easily visualize myself as a ninety-year-old man jogging lithely in a local park.

So can we reprogram ourselves to think differently and appreciate the world? To learn more about the subject, I interviewed Ho'oponopono expert Mabel Katz. As I mentioned above, she describes Ho'oponopono as "the easiest way" to live, and she wrote a book series with the same title (*The Easiest Way*[4]). Mabel is an Argentine Jew who worked as an accountant for much of her life, and she was married with two healthy children. She had enough money to buy a house, cars, and some of life's luxurious pleasures, but she found she was not happy. She allowed the little things in life to make her angry, and she was constantly reacting to the turmoil caused by her children, her career, and her family.

It turns out that it is very difficult to change the world around you. The world is stochastic, complex, and arbitrary. There are too many factors to take into consideration and too many forces which you cannot control. It is very difficult to convince other people to change their manner of behavior. It is much easier to change yourself. This is the concept of one-hundred percent responsibility—the commitment to accept total responsibility for how you feel and how you react to the world.

Because of how she felt, Mabel pursued a new quest to find her spiritual self. She started reading books and going to seminars. She went to a sweat lodge, performed rebirthing, and took part in many other rituals[4, page 86]. By chance, she found Ho'oponopono, and she ended up under the tutelage of the well-known Dr. Ihaleakalá Hew Len. Throughout the rest of this chapter, her words are in italics.

I started my search because of anger. I was a very angry, frustrated person—unhappy even though I had everything that you think you need in order to be happy. My oldest son one day acted as a mirror because he talked to me in the angry way I used to talk to him, and so I saw myself. I actually woke up. I realized that he learned from me. Our kids don't listen; they observe. I said, "Mabel, you have to do something." I thought happiness was to be healthy, to have material things, security, university titles, a house, a husband, and kids.

Mabel took the leap of faith and gave up her career as an accountant, believing that teaching Ho'oponopono was something that she was meant to do. When she transitioned, she was not entirely financially secure, but everything worked out for her. She now has five published books, and she travels around the world giving lectures and guiding retreats. She has been to Madrid, Budapest, India, Bucharest, Mt. Shasta, Belgrade, Israel, Asia, Cancun, and many other places to popularize Ho'oponopono. When I met her, I immediately saw the reason for her success: she has a deep seated and genuine happiness and confidence that is truly rare. I got the feeling that she knew something that I did not know, and I started asking questions.

One principle of Ho'oponopono is that you are responsible for attracting things in your life. If you are attracting negative things, look within yourself and not outside of yourself. Do not allow a disease or anything external to determine your self-worth. Do not let your state of mind become too dependent on a doctor, a friend, a family member, or a politician. Say to yourself, "I'm sorry; please forgive me for whatever is in me that created this." This is about empowerment, not culpability. It is about taking back the locus of control for yourself and denying it to the world. This is in its very essence an optimistic worldview because it means that you will see yourself as an agent rather than a victim.

The secret to happiness is not looking outside or looking for more. It is developing our capacity to love and enjoy ourselves more[4, page 103]. We attach so much to other people and to conditions. We are dependent, and that is very frustrating to everybody. You have to be able to be with yourself, to love yourself, and to accept yourself. What is important is what you think of you and not what other people think of you. When you take one-hundred percent responsibility, you make relationships more harmonious because you're not blaming others or needing to be right or demanding the last word. Ho'oponopono helped me to realize that I don't know anything and that everything is a blessing. That gives you a lot of peace of mind, and if you are at peace, everything can be solved.

Connected with this is the concept of limiting expectations and requirements of the world around us. If we demand too much of the world, it is likely to disappoint us. If we are more willing to roll with the punches, we become more adaptive. This is similar to the accommodative coping style discussed in Chapter Five, but Mabel adds her own twist. Consider the following tale which is taken from a fable and is also described in Mabel's book[4, page 49-52].

In a small medieval village, there was once a very poor old man who was supported by the hard labor of his only son. He owned a beautiful white horse which was the envy of the local townspeople. One day, a wealthy lord offered the old man a generous sum of money for the horse, but the old man refused because he saw the horse as a member of his family. The townspeople said to him, "You are a fool. What is a pretty horse to an old man? The money could have supported you in your old age." The man replied, "You judge too quickly. Say only that I did not sell my horse. No one knows what the future holds."

A few months later, the white horse went missing, and everyone presumed it was taken by thieves. The townspeople said to him, "Poor old man. It would have been better had you sold it. What a shame!" He again replied stoically, "Let us not assume. We can only say that my horse has gone missing. Everything else is your judgment. If it is bad luck or good, I do not know because this is merely a fragment. Who knows what will happen tomorrow." The townspeople mocked his foolishness and pitied his misfortune. However, in a fortnight, the white horse returned and brought with him a beautiful black horse that quickly became the talk of the town. The townspeople said, "You were right, old man! Your bad luck has turned to good!"

The old man replied, "Once again, you go too far. Say only that my white horse has returned and brought with it a black horse. This is fact, but it is only a fragment of my life—only a single sentence of a book." The villagers thought the old man was a bit crazy, but they were happy for him nonetheless. Soon after, the old man's son began to train the black horse, and he accidentally fell and broke his arm. The locals again convened and said, "You were right again, old man. It was misfortune after all. The black horse was a curse, and now your only son can no longer support you. You are poorer than ever."

"You are obsessed with judging," said the old man. "Do not get carried away. Let us say that my son has fallen and broken his arm. We do not know if this is a misfortune or a blessing. This is only a fragment—only one step in the recipe. Life comes in small bits and pieces, and from these pieces we cannot judge the whole."

Shortly after this, the country declared war on a neighboring state and conscripted all the young men in the village to the army. They spared the old man's son because of his injury. The commoners lamented, "You were right again, old man. They have taken our sons from us to fight a hopeless war. Your son will recover with time, but ours may never return."

Again, the old man scoffed. "You are still judging. Nobody knows what will come of this war. Say only that your sons have been forced to join the army and that my son has not been forced. Only God knows if this is bad luck or good."

The old man teaches us to take the world as it comes. There will be twists and turns throughout our lives, and we never know where a particular fork in the road will lead us. Mabel encourages us to "trust and let go"[4, page 76]. We must "allow ourselves to be surprised by the universe"[4, page 114]. Do not do this because you think it is metaphysically accurate. The reality is that the world is cold, harsh, and brutal. Do this despite reality. Do this because it is practical. Do this because it will prevent you from becoming depressed and will force you to see things in a positive light and to make the best of your situation. Mabel encourages us to view obstacles in life as opportunities to improve ourselves. I actually looked back at the quote I composed for my high school yearbook, and I found a similar piece of wisdom. I was only seventeen at the time, but I wrote something which is still meaningful to me today:

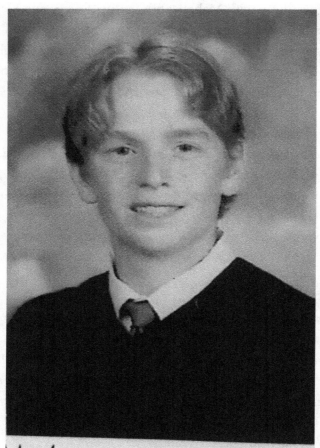

Brandon Beaber

"Stones are the obstacles
on the path of life. Some
trip over them, some walk
around them, and some walk
over them." Dont toss
these stones aside, for
they are made of gold.

This goes along with Mabel's philosophy of accepting life's hardships. She believes resisting causes great suffering. She says, "What you resist persists." Instead of fighting with the world, fight with yourself. Learn to accept yourself and who you are even if this means you have an illness or a disability.

You are not alone. You are being protected and guided. This is right even if it doesn't look right, so you just go with it. You observe it, and you say, "Thank you." You don't give it the power. Moment by moment, you are choosing who you are going to give power to. It's not like I don't have problems or that I'm completely healthy. I also have my challenges, but I don't give them the power. When you start seeing the results, you really start seeing the power that you have, and you realize where that power is and how to use it.

I learned to trust uncertainty and to live very much in the present. I don't make a lot of plans, but I learned to trust, and amazing things happen. I live a different kind of life because I learned that the power resides in me and that I create my life, and I am responsible for it. I trust completely, so I live an uncertain life. I don't need security. I know that I will be taken care of and that I will be in the right place at the right time with the right people.

This ability to trust and focus on the present is critical for people with MS. If you are thinking too much about the history of your illness and the disabilities you have already acquired, it is difficult to be adaptive and to look forward. If you are too fearful of the future, it is impossible to enjoy life and the abilities you do have. Could Dr. Bhat succeed as a psychiatrist if he focused on the past? Could Dr. Spitz pursue a stroke fellowship if she were overwhelmed with concerns about a future flare hindering her career? They are both forced to live in the present if they want to thrive. Of course, there is a balance we must find. Some people are so nonchalant that they neglect themselves and worsen their condition. What is underappreciated is that it is equally dangerous to be overly vigilant and single-minded, turning an illness into your entire identity.

> *I can be happy, and I can be at peace even if I have a disease. The disease will depend on how I approach it. If I see myself as a victim, I am resisting. If we depend on other people's acceptance, caring, or attention, we learn to depend on other people when everything we need is inside of us. I know that doctors say there is a difference in the progression of an illness or the progression of a cure if people believe or if they don't. We have power in our thoughts. If you change your thoughts, you change everything. If I am sick, my goal is not to be healed. My goal is to be at peace even if I'm sick. If you're at peace and you're happy, everything comes to you. If you resist, fear the disease, and see yourself as a victim, you're doing exactly the opposite. That's how powerful we are. Everything is a blessing and is showing up in your life to show you have something important to do or that you need to wake up.*

What Mabel says here sounds too idealistic but cannot be discounted. Sometimes, illness can have unexpectedly positive effects. When I was fellow training in neuroimmunology, I attended a conference funded by Don Tykeson, a well-known businessman and donor to MS charities. Don Tykeson was himself diagnosed with MS at age thirty, and he attributes the diagnosis to much of his business success, going so far as to refer to MS as "his old friend." The fear of becoming disabled made him more aggressive, impatient, and diligent in his business pursuits. Tykeson launched a successful broadcasting and cable television enterprise, allowing him to enrich not just himself but also the MS community at large with his philanthropic endeavors. His own words show us the positive effect that MS had on his life:

"I knew I needed to be bold and take some risks; in that sense, MS has served me well" —Don Tykeson[8]

One can easily find a hundred similar examples. Oprah Winfrey, a victim of sexual abuse, was inspired by her experience to discuss her past publicly and to help others[9]. Ray Charles became a world-famous musician despite becoming blind in his youth due to glaucoma[10]. It is said that his blindness forced him to utilize his memory for music and to develop his gift of perfect pitch[11]. Prior to being diagnosed with Lou Gehrig's disease at age twenty-one, Stephen Hawking was "laid back and bored with life," but the illness changed his mindset, launching his legendary career in theoretical physics[12]. When something unfortunate befalls you, try to think of the event as a wake-up call or a kick in the rear. Think of how you can turn your misfortune into a bonanza, and this mindset may turn into a self-fulfilling prophecy. This is analogous to the "broaden and build" model described by Frederickson which we discussed in Chapter Three.

That being said, it is difficult to avoid dwelling on our troubles in life. This is the nature of our minds. We analyze things, looking for patterns and explanations. This is useful in many aspects of life, but according to Mabel, we must suppress the intellect to an extent or it will take over our lives. What she proposes is a very counterintuitive idea because the intellect serves us so well in so many contexts. Abstract thinking differentiates us from the animals, and we learn about its importance from a young age. However, it is a double-edged sword. We have to know when to quiet down our analytical mind when it is causing us more harm than good. Remember the lesson of the old man: events in life may not be as straight forward as we realize, and the assumptions we make—even about our own desires and preferences—may not be accurate.

The fight that I invite people to pursue is the fight of letting go of the intellect that is always talking...always having opinions and judgments. Every time we worry, we are saying, "God, I know more than you. I can do it alone." This is the intellect that you think knows and has the university titles and is very smart. You have to become humble and realize you don't know anything.

This is another principle of Ho'oponopono—that our memories and programs are toxic, and we need to "clean" them from our minds. Memories derive from our experiences and childhood traumas. Some of them are even passed down through generations. They are algorithmic procedures, and they put us on autopilot, making us act without thinking and making us feel what we are "supposed" to feel. We even unconsciously give these programs to our children. When we think about what we want for our children, we are quick to list that we want them to be healthy, attractive, successful, and fertile. Strangely, we leave off this list that we want them to be happy. We somehow view this as less important, or we wrongly believe happiness will automatically accompany these other things. In reality, they correlate very poorly with happiness. In this way, we are almost addicted to these programs and memories, and we can become addicted to the pain and suffering they cause.

Einstein said the definition of insanity is doing the same thing over and over again but expecting different results. We are a very insane species. However, Mabel believes we can clean our minds of these negative memories and programs by using the mantras of Ho'oponopono along with other techniques. By simply saying "thank you," we are accepting what comes to us in life and not giving power to the memories. If we do this and make ourselves happier, all the other things we desire for ourselves and our children will tend to come naturally. Happy people are more productive. They attract friends and allies. They are more resilient when things go awry.

You don't need to feel it working or anything. You just need to stop the left hemisphere and its opinions and judgments. You want to be present. When you worry, you are worrying about what will happen to you in a month or a year from now. How are you going to survive? Where is your money coming from? Who is going to take care of you? That's all the future. All you have to be is in the present, and in the present, you have everything you need. So moment by moment, you're saying, "thank you" and "I love you." When a doctor gives you a diagnosis, are you going to call your relatives and tell them that a terrible thing happened? Or, are you going to say, "Thank you; thank you; thank you. God, I'll give it to you. I don't have any clue what to do here. This is too much for me. This is really scary." I'm not saying you're going to be cured because I don't know what is right, and I don't know what kind of decisions you are going to make. I do know that everything is possible when I let go.

Of course, it is perfectly natural and expected to reach out to your loved ones after receiving a terrifying diagnosis. The desire to grieve, vent, and search for comfort are natural human emotions, and we should not criticize them. However, Mabel encourages us to do something different and counterintuitive. She believes we should accept our fate and erase negative thoughts through the process of cleaning.

She recommends various techniques for cleaning the mind. One of them is to use the mantras. When something happens to you in life, be it positive or negative, say "thank you" in your mind. Accept what comes to you without judgment or complaint, and try to see things optimistically. Foster this habit by setting aside a specific time each day or week to think about what you can be thankful for. When you interact with people, try to say, "I love you" in your mind. Think of the things you love about the other person, and try to see that person in a very positive light. People will recognize your attitude and energy, and this will pay dividends. The musician Ozzy Osbourne understands this, and he once said, "I have a genuine love affair with my audience. When I'm on stage, they're not privileged to see me. It's a privilege for me to see them." Say "I love you" to yourself as a reminder that you unconditionally and completely love yourself just the way you are. According to Joe Vitale, "Loving yourself is the greatest way to improve yourself, and as you improve yourself, you improve your world"[5].

If something negative happens in your life, say "I'm sorry" in your mind even if you are not at fault. Say, "I'm sorry for whatever it is in me that created this." Sometimes, it is necessary to "let go" instead of trying to think about what you can do to help the situation, and when you are in a dispute with someone, try to take at least some responsibility for the conflict.

Life is certain to bring you stress and anxiety at times, so Mabel suggests a few relaxation techniques. One approach is ha breathing, a Hawaiian breathing technique. Start by sitting in a relaxed position, and close your eyes. Slow down your breathing, and with each inhalation, count to seven in your head. Then, hold the inhalation and silently count to seven again. Next, breath out slowly, again counting to seven throughout the exhalation. Repeat this routine a total of seven times. During the process, focus only on your breathing and allow the exercise to clear your mind.

Another technique is to use a glass of water as a symbol for the conflict in your life. In the morning, fill a glass of water three quarters full. Let this water represent your day-to-day troubles or whatever is occupying your conscious mind at the moment. Every morning and every evening, dump out the water and replace it. If during the day you experience something particularly troubling, you can change the water to calm yourself. As you dump out the water, imagine your thoughts and memories being transmuted and replaced with a clean slate representing "the state of zero." Mabel teaches many other techniques, and you if you are interested, you can read her books or go to her website at www.mabelkatz.com.

Mabel did not get into Ho'oponopono because she thought the ideology was logically sound. Some traditions are hokey, and she well knows this. Ho'oponopono just empirically works for her, and she has been undeniably happier since taking up the practice. She had been practicing the principles for many years when Dr. Ihaleakalá Hew Len retired, and he allowed her to take over his seminars and students. She was not financially secure at the time, and she did not know if everything would work out, but it felt right to her, so she took the leap of faith.

I try to apply the principles of Ho'oponopono to my own life as well. I read a few of Mabel's books and attended one of her seminars (which I would highly recommend). Sometimes, I will become frustrated at work when patients are difficult or require extra time. I try to think to myself, "I love you." I think about what makes this person unique and about the contribution this person makes to the world. I think to myself, "Thank you" for giving me the opportunity to be part of your medical care and to practice my craft. I try not to react negatively when things go haywire. Patients are late or noncompliant with treatment. Coworkers are discourteous at times. Nights on call can be busy. Diagnostic tests do not get done or treatments are unsuccessful. These are things I should accept as part of being a doctor. I try to think of these as normal and unavoidable, and I realize that it is I who must change, not the world around me.

I have applied the principles in my personal life as well. Instead of complaining, I say "thank you" for all that I appreciate. I say "I love you" genuinely and passionately. When there is a disagreement, I try to think about changing myself rather than changing the other person. My wife and I do ha breathing for relaxation and inner peace.

In the context of MS, there is no doubt the principles of Ho'oponopono have much to offer. People with MS are under a tremendous amount of stress, and they need ways to manage this.

They also would benefit from the self-love, self-responsibility, and optimistic thinking promoted by the philosophy. Sometimes, we need more than just a series of practical suggestions; we need a life doctrine to ground us. In this way, Ho'oponopono serves almost as a religion, providing a framework for implementing sustained changes in mindset and values. You may not become a dedicated Ho'oponopono practitioner like Mabel, but understanding her principles and applying some of her suggestions could make a big difference in your life.

CHAPTER SEVEN REFERENCES

1. Fahlgren E, Nima AA, Archer T, Garcia D. Person-centered osteopathic practice: patients' personality (body, mind, and soul) and health (ill-being and well-being. *PeerJ* 2015 Oct 27;3:e1349.
2. Kretzer K. Integrating a CAM Therapeutic Strategy for Hypertension. *Am J Nurse Pract* 2011 Nov;15(11-12):48-52.
3. Ito KL. Ho'oponopono, "to make right": Hawaiian conflict resolution and metaphor in the construction of a family therapy. *Cult Med Psychiatry* 1985 Jun;9(2):201-17.
4. Katz M. The Easiest Way: Solve Your Problems and Take the Road to Love, Happiness, Wealth and the Life of Your Dreams. Your Business Press, January 25, 2010.
5. Vitale J, Ihaleakala HL. Zero Limits. Wiley, 2007.
6. Carnegie D. *How to Win Friends & Influence People.* Simon & Schuster, October 1, 1998.
7. Gehrig L. Farewell Address. July 4, 1939. Available at http://www.lougehrig.com/about/farewell.html.
8. The National MS Society. Don Tykeson. Available at http://www.nationalmssociety.org/Living-Well-With-MS/Personal-Stories/Tributes/Don-Tykeson.
9. Winfrey L. Praise from All Corners for New Talk Show Host. *Syracuse Herald Journal*, September 9, 1986, p. 44.
10. Graham E. Obituary: Ray Charles (1930 – 2004). *Bohème Magazine*, 2004.
11. Ray Charles Biography. Encyclopedia of world biography. Available at http://www.notablebiographies.com/Ch-Co/Charles-Ray.html
12. Kendrick D. Illness put Hawking on path to greatness. January 28, 2001

CHAPTER 8:
MIGUEL HERNANDEZ

"If you're going to kick authority
in the teeth, you might as well use two feet."
—Keith Richards, *Keith Richards: In His Own Words*

MIGUEL HERNANDEZ IS a thirty-one-year-old with re-lapsing MS who is legally blind. He lost his vision quickly and unexpectedly while early in his personal development at the budding age of twenty-one. Even before he became ill, his life was a rollercoaster of poor decision making, drug abuse, and crime. He started smoking weed at age nine and was doing hard drugs regularly in junior high school. When I listen to his story, I am amazed he avoided incarceration or worse during his youth. His history reminds me of how differently people experience childhood. He and I both grew up in Los Angeles within ten miles of each other, but we could not have had a more different upbringing. Aside from his vision, he is only minimally affected by the disease, but even the simplest things which we all take for granted give him trouble now. However, despite MS (or perhaps because of MS), he has turned his life around. He now works full time, is engaged to a woman he loves, and is an active volunteer with big dreams for the future. This is a story of how conflict interacts with and shapes character and resilience. It teaches us that resilience is found and forged in unexpected places and in all walks of life.

Miguel's mother, the youngest of nine children, is from Guatemala, and his father is from El Salvador. They came to the United States in the mid-1980s, and Miguel was born in 1987. He came into the world with an umbilical cord wrapped around his neck, and doctors pushed him back into the uterus and performed an emergency C-section, but no complications ensued. His parents tell the story dramatically, saying that he was born "dead," but after that harrowing beginning, he was a normal child without developmental problems. His mother has a proud Mayan heritage, and his father also shares a traditional Amerindian mindset with an emphasis on a close-knit family, hard work, and self-sufficiency. When they arrived in LaFayette, a mostly Hispanic city near downtown Los Angeles, they were given nothing and had nothing. Miguel has a tremendous respect and admiration for his parents and their background.

They're very conservative and private. They are independent as I was never raised with food stamps. We didn't have anything. My father was so proud; he would say, "I can do it. I can do it." He raised us like that. Many moms are in the welfare office waiting for money and that sort of stuff. My parents didn't do that; they are hard-working people. My parents gave me that. I'm a hard worker as well, and I like to work. I don't like to be a sloppy lazy one just expecting a paycheck; I'm gonna work to get my paychecks.

His parents always eschewed accepting handouts or looking for outside assistance, more due to stubborn pride than political philosophy. In 1992, they had a daughter, Miguel's only sibling. His mother got a job in a Guess jeans factory, sewing zippers into jeans and the like. She would get paid by the pound, and she would frequently bring jeans home and work late to support Miguel and his younger sister.

My mom was wicked. I just remember a ridiculous amount of bags. I would come home and think, "What are all these trash bags?" That was all the linen—all the jeans that my mom was sewing.

Miguel's father works for a contractor. Although he has no formal training, he is a wizard with electrical work, plumbing, and other home and industrial maintenance issues. Despite being a fifty-nine-year-old diabetic with a bad left knee, he works long hours and is always out of the door by 6:30 AM. Miguel learned this trade from a young age, and his father would bring him to work as a form of punishment. He picked up both the technical skills and the mindset of a fastidious blue-collar worker. He could later impress friends and girlfriends with his ability to fix things around their homes. The experience encouraged an autonomous mindset—the belief people should do everything for themselves if they are capable and learn to do new things if they are incapable.

Years later, his mother got a job a Levy's restaurant at the Staples Center, the stadium where the Los Angeles Lakers play. She works as a cook, and at one point, she dislocated her right shoulder carrying a heavy food tray. She was in terrible pain but did not miss a single day of work because she needed to maintain a certain number of hours to get health insurance for her family. The work was hard and required sacrifices, but there were rewards as well. They lived a simple but dignified life and were never destitute or dependent on anyone else. They eventually went through the proper channels and became American citizens.

His parents spoke English very poorly when they first came to the country, but Miguel had a good early educational experience and was somewhat precocious. He was reading in kindergarten, and he had an encouraging teacher who recognized his talent and referred him to a magnet school in the San Fernando Valley.

Sesame Street taught me English. I just remember Mr. Carrejo who was my kindergarten teacher. I had chicken pox, and he would come to the house because he liked the fact that I would read, and he would bring books to read. I remember that.

His academic progress overjoyed his parents even though they were illiterate in English and would not have known the difference between reading and confabulation. They saw the value of a quality American education, and they wanted a better and easier life for Miguel than they had for themselves. They encouraged his independence and even gave him a spending allowance to help him learn to save and manage money. He received love, a stable home, and good values from his parents. They tried to carve out a niche of stability in a crazy world, but this did not stop Miguel from rebelling. It is hard to instill traditional values in your children when a corrupting environment surrounds them, and you do not have the cultural insight to comprehend it.

One problem was that Miguel lost his local circle of friends and now had to take a long bus ride to school every day. As he socialized less outside of school, he spent more and more time with friends during school hours. Unlike many kids, he did not like staying inside and playing video games but rather preferred skateboarding, soccer, and just wandering around. He would skip school or sneak out at night to meet up with his friends for sports, ice cream, or burgers. Initially, his parents saw no cause for concern as he maintained all outward appearances of being a good kid, and they had little concept of this form of delinquency. When he was in 4th grade, a friend's older sister introduced him to marijuana, and he gladly obliged. A new experience quickly became a regular habit, and he fell into a crowd where weed was always available. He became argumentative and defiant. His academic performance deteriorated, and in the 7th grade, they downgraded him from the magnet program to the general education track.

I was also a pyro for a while. We'd have candles, and I would just set things on fire. Accidents would happen—like I'm playing with fire, and then "whoosh," a curtain sets on fire. That's a major accident because, "Oh no! How am I gonna hide that?" Heh heh. We used to steal. We used to shoplift and stuff. We were really young; it started with sunflower seeds and then beer, food, chips, and that kind of stuff.

They would usually get away with it, and even when caught, they would simply return the items or run away. His parents never found out, and accordingly, there were never any disciplinary consequences. The mischief was for fun rather than greed. His family was poor but never penniless, and because of his allowance, he had more spending cash than most of his friends. At around age twelve or thirteen, he graduated from weed to cocaine, meth, and other stimulants. He did not have to search for drugs; they surrounded him. He remembers being chastised at one point by his friends for doing cocaine but refusing to do harder drugs that were available at the time. Still, he grew long hair and fit right in with the stoners. It became a major part of his social identity and his day-to-day life.

Snorting through your right nostril goes to your body as you take it in. Going through your left nostril, it hits your head. It goes to your brain and comes back down. I feel that is how I messed up my system because from a young age, I always went through my left because if you want to get high, get high—you know? I started with coke and then went on to other drugs, mixing other drugs and cooking other shit. I feel that I gave myself MS like that, but it's a theory. How can it be proven? Drugs are bad, period. I learned that. I learned my lesson.

His comments about nostril laterality and the connection between drug use and MS are dubious, but this is beside the point. His academic success spiraled from superior to average to marginal to miserable. High in class much of the time he was not ditching school, he failed to graduate middle school. He had to attend summer school to make up for lost time which quickly became a regular tradition. He did not care about school and had no long-term goals or ambitions. It was all about fun, alcohol, drugs, and later, girls. He focused on social standing, money, rebellion, and short-term gratification. In high school, he had a transient interest in drama, improv, and writing, and teachers noticed his talent, but he did not have the focus or diligence to materialize these skills. The only classes where he performed well were drama and stage crew—the former because of his interest and the latter because of the handiness and hard work he had learned from his father. His parents were mostly left in the dark until they would attend parent-teacher conferences and learn that their son had not been in school for weeks.

When they learned about this and his other troubles, it devastated them. They did not understand. They had worked so hard, fed him well, kept him safe, and taught him good values. He was to be the privileged amongst the underprivileged. His sister never had any similar problems despite the same environment.

Miguel went to adult school summer after summer. He remembers taking a 9th grade class the summer before 12th grade because he had failed so many classes. Taking up to six classes during a single summer, he got through largely by forging assignments and cramming for exams. He passed despite an incredible lack of work ethic, except for brief spurts before final exams. His only motivation was to prove to his parents that he could get a high school diploma. Older high school students and even young adults dominated these classes, so he began to hang out with an older crowd which led to harder drugs and more serious criminal activity. As time passed, he focused more and more on making money. He got a job at Rubio's Fresh Mexican Grill at age seventeen while still in high school.

He supplemented his income from Rubio's by selling drugs and stolen items along with a series of robberies perpetrated by him and a small group of friends. They would target disenfranchised immigrants working for cash, threatening their victims with a knife or simply surrounding them and forcing them to hand over their money earned from a long day of manual labor. Their victims did not have bank accounts, and they would often carry around rent money. Again, Miguel did not truly need the money except to buy drugs. He was simply reckless, greedy, and opportunistic. He was never punished or even discovered. It was easy money, and with money came drugs and girls.

I used to get laid a lot, but it was because of the drugs. I used to sell drugs to bitches left and right. I had what I would call dopehead sluts.

Despite the vulgar terminology, Miguel sees himself as a "hopeless romantic," and he saw himself in this way even back then. He did not truly want one-night stands or short-term flings with addicts. He wanted a conservative girl to show off to his parents. He wanted a stable job, a white picket fence, a wife, and a family. His conservative upbringing never completely left him, and he still had many of his parents' values, but he became entrenched in self-defeating behavior. He realizes retrospectively he was not doing the things or living the lifestyle that would attract the girl he desired.

During prom night, he suddenly realized he had no genuine friends. All of his connections were through drugs and crime. He was not in any pictures, and he had neither a date nor a group of friends with which to socialize. No one was close or loyal to him; he had just become the guy people go to when they want to buy drugs. He sold ecstasy to a couple who promptly left, but aside from that, he hardly talked to anyone. After dancing with some girls and dropping acid, he woke up in Echo Park. It was at this point he had a moment of reflection. He stopped doing drugs cold turkey, and he ceased all criminal activity. The lifestyle had grown weary. He now saw these behaviors as an illness to purge, and the catharsis was liberating. He did not become a saint overnight as he continued to drink heavily for many years. However, he stayed away from hard drugs, stopped committing crimes, and cut ties with many of his less scrupulous acquaintances. He finished high school on time, and his graduation was a moment of great pride for him and his parents.

After high school, he worked at Rubio's for a period, and then he got a new job in the UCLA dining commons at Panda Express where he made $1.50 more an hour. He did not mind the work, but being in that environment made him realize that he had greater ambitions in life.

It hit me because I was serving lunch to beautiful women and college students, and I was like, "What the fuck am I doing here?" I'm around

a bunch of spics and shit, and this is all we can do here in the States?
I'mma go to school.

And so he did. He enrolled at Santa Monica College (SMC), a junior college in West Los Angeles ten miles from LaFayette. He had only missed the fall semester, so he was more or less a typical college freshman. SMC provided a supportive environment, and he majored in English, developing a love for literature and poetry. Indeed, his professors found him to be a talented writer. In his eyes, the beauty of writing is having the power to affect someone's emotions, positively or negatively. However, impatience accompanied his ambition. He wanted to taste success as quickly as possible, and he had no role models or mentors to encourage him to stay the course. Furthermore, he was always more comfortable in the work setting than in the academic setting, so he quit SMC to work at an orthopedics office.

He started out as a file clerk and later became an office clerk. He would help with the logistics of the office, address random maintenance problems, fix furniture, and do other odd jobs to help the doctors and staff. Productive, skilled, and hard-working, he made $13 an hour which was a lot for a young man with modest tastes living with his parents. He was always a saver rather than a spender. He would recycle old items from the street, wear simple clothing, and solve problems himself without hiring professionals. With his drug habit squashed, he had plenty of discretionary income and was saving up a nest egg.

Though he did not know it at the time, his symptoms of MS began in his late teenage years. He never would have suspected anything was seriously wrong, but he began having problems with his right shoulder. He would have tightness and muscle spasms. He would wake up, and his right shoulder and arm would lock out with his elbow flexed and his biceps tightened. It was a painful experience, temporarily immobilizing him and thrusting him out of bed, screaming in pain. This type of symptom is well-known in MS and has been called a "paroxysmal symptom." These events with dystonic flexion of muscles are known as flexor spasms. We can treat them with muscle relaxants or seizure medications like carbamazepine. He attributed the episodes to prior drug use, and they later resolved.

In 2008, he developed discomfort in his left eye, but there were no changes in vision, and the sensation soon resolved spontaneously. In 2009, he was hit by a car while bicycling near the corner of 3rd and Figueroa, and he was thrown off his bike onto the pavement. He had no injuries, but thereafter, he noted a slight imbalance when walking due to a subtle incoordination of his left leg. Retrospectively, he thinks this incoordination may have existed beforehand and may have caused the accident to occur in the first place. The symptom persisted for a few weeks but then resolved as quickly as it came on.

He was doing well working for the medical practice, but he knew deep down he needed more education to accomplish his long-term goals. He quit his job in 2009 and went to Los Angeles City College (LACC) to study psychology and human resources. Unfortunately, he did not have the same experience at LACC that he had at SMC. SMC is a reputable junior college with a high transfer rate to well-known four-year universities such as UCLA and USC. At LACC, Miguel felt the teachers and students were not as motivated. The school's resources were inferior, and the culture was different. Because of this and the desire for a quicker route to a career, he dropped out and attended Associated Technical College (ATC), a well-known trade school.

While he was attending LACC and ATC, Miguel made new friends to replace the connections he had in high school with drug dealers, addicts, and vandals. He was a punk rocker for a while, but he later fell into a crowd of urban anarchists. These were well-educated people with prestigious degrees who chose to live an alternative lifestyle in a tight-knit and philanthropic community. The group was Food Not Bombs, a collective started in 1980 which stages anti-war protests and provides food to the needy with an all-volunteer work-force[1]. They would get unused produce and baked goods from farms and businesses, prepare food on site, and serve meals to the homeless or anyone who was hungry and wanting. Miguel loved the community and the feeling of independence. He became a regular volunteer, and it gave him a great sense of satisfaction. He even became voluntarily homeless for a while to truly live the anarchist lifestyle, sleeping on the streets in downtown near skid row on cardboard dispensed by an Asian woman who was a friend of the community.

At first, he was in it for the friendships and the lifestyle, but he also values the political ideology: charity, self-sufficiency, and opposition to war. He became a "VIP" after a while, and he even gave a PowerPoint presentation about the organization at a city hall meeting, showing pictures of the gatherings to city officials. The organization would clash with law enforcement because they would attract large numbers of homeless people in concentrated areas. During one such clash, SWAT vans approached the scene, and Miguel and his friends took off running, leaving all the food behind. They later found out that the vans were empty, and it was all for show.

He would shower at LACC and use their lockers while he was a student there. He would get around using his bus pass he obtained through school. From his perspective, he was living like a king and had all he needed. When he transferred to ATC, he wanted to be a surgical technician, an assistant to the surgeon in the operating room. The career is exciting, fast paced, and relatively high paying. He had all the prerequisites. He was young, energetic, hard-working, and good with his hands. Everything was going well until May 2010 when the big accident happened.

He had just acquired and refurbished a new bicycle—a beautiful GT that he was excited to take for a ride with his friends. At 6th and Figueroa, his brakes gave out, and he lost control, running through a red light, turning into a driveway, and flipping forward head-first into a wall. He was unconscious for eleven hours and woke up in LA County Hospital with countless injuries including a fractured skull and missing teeth. He was delirious from pain, morphine, and post-concussive syndrome. A CT scan of the head revealed no major intracranial injuries, but the scan coincidentally found lesions suspicious for MS. They considered the diagnosis of MS instantly, but this was either not disclosed to him, or he does not remember hearing about it due to concussion-induced anterograde amnesia. At one point, he was well enough to go to the bathroom, and he looked in the mirror to find he had lost many of his teeth in the accident. He remembers a gruesome face looking back at him.

I went back into the bed, and I was just screaming, and I was like, "I need morphine!"

He recovered enough to be discharged, but shortly afterwards, he developed optic neuritis in both of his eyes. First, there was pain in his left eye, and his vision became blurry. He recalls he could not look up with his eyes because this would worsen his pain. Soon after this, the condition attacked his right eye and profoundly impaired his overall vision. There was a brief period of denial where he attributed his poor vision to the head injury. In addition, he saw little point in seeing doctors because all doctors do is deliver bad news. However, the symptoms were dramatic and unambiguous, so he went back to the emergency room and was quickly hooked up with the neurology clinic at County Hospital. They listened to the rest of his history, put the pieces together, and a spinal tap confirmed an official diagnosis of MS. He could not help but think MS resulted from bad karma from prior indiscretions.

I went to a room with a big 'ol screen, and they showed me my brain, and the first thing that came to my mind was, "I did this. I know I did this." They said, "You have a disease," and I thought I had AIDS or something. I was like, "No! Don't tell me this now. I'm blind with AIDS!" She explained it to me, but I'm not a doctor; I don't speak medical. MS? At first, I thought she was talking about a gang. The doctor had told me, "There's a possibility that you will get your vision back." I remember I screamed, "When! Give me a date! Dammit!" Is it gonna get better in a year? Is it gonna get better in forty? I was like, "Doc; you can't do this to me!"

To this day, Miguel has relatively low health literacy. I have patients who are practically experts in MS and could quote research studies and discuss drug side effects with incredible sophistication. Miguel has neither the background nor the interest to do this. He is a pragmatic person. What do I have? What do I need to do? Will I get better? Unfortunately, no one could answer the last question, and he believed for months his vision might return. He actually did improve somewhat. At its nadir, his vision was so poor that he could hardly see shapes and could not comfortably cross a busy intersection. After many years, he has finger-counting vision only in the left eye and 20/400 vision in the right eye. In other words, in his "good" right eye, he can see at twenty feet what a normal person can see at 400 feet. The giant "E" at the top of a Snellen chart in your doctor's office represents 20/200 vision. This "E" would be too small for Miguel to see. His left eye is even worse than this, so most of his functional vision is from the right eye. Legal blindness is defined as visual acuity of 20/200 or worse in the better eye[2], and Miguel clearly meets this criterion. If you are knowledgeable about MS, you might wonder to yourself, does Miguel actually have the disease? Could he have another condition which more typically causes severe bilateral visual loss such as neuromyelitis optica or Leber's hereditary optic neuropathy? Take my word for it; he definitely has MS. Developing early severe vision loss in both eyes is uncommon in MS, but it can occur. Furthermore, Miguel's MRI scans show lesions which are highly typical of MS:

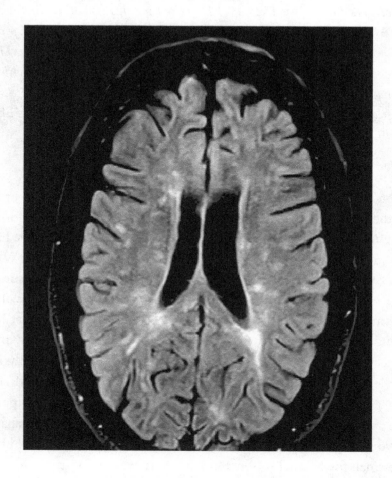

Figure 1: An axial T2 FLAIR MRI at the level of the lateral ventricles showing typical MS lesions.

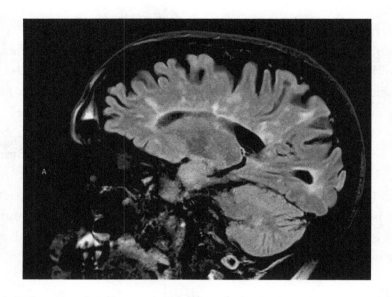

Figure 2: A parasagittal T2 FLAIR MRI near the corpus callosum showing typical MS lesions resembling a "picket fence" (a well-known finding in MS)

It might surprise you to see that Miguel has fairly extensive lesions despite relatively low disability aside from his visual loss. This is not unusual because the MRI scan does not tell us much about the function of the diseased tissue. Much of this abnormal tissue may be riddled with demyelination or inflammation, but it may function well. In fact, the correlation between brain lesion burden and disability is quite poor[3]. Miguel's case is an example of "clinicoradiological dissociation"—a dissociation between radiologic findings and clinical findings[4].

Miguel tried to go back to ATC for a period with the hope he would scrape by and pretend nothing was wrong, but it was futile. He could not read his textbooks let alone draw blood or do anything technical. He finally broke down and told his professors what was wrong in private, and he later dropped out. He was devastated. After finally getting on the path to a stable career the

American dream his parents wanted for him, something so sto-chastic and arbitrary derailed him. He was five months into a nine-month program when he left. He had no choice but to move back in with his parents, lacking both his vision and a purpose in life. For close to a year, he was depressed, unproductive, and feeling sorry for himself, waiting to see if he would improve. This was not the neurovegetative depression with melancholy and lethargy from which Sandra Orozco suffered; it was a profound disappointment with where he was in life. The doctors also treated him for anxiety and post-traumatic stress disorder. When he was stressed or angry, his vision would temporarily worsen, mimicking a relapse and in-ducing paranoia.

> *I couldn't really do it anymore. I got sad. I got depressed. Here you are; you aren't doing shit. Then, the year passed, and I accepted it. I'm like, "I'm blind." I'm stuck. There ain't nothing else that's gonna happen. Remember those commercials where they say don't do drugs because you're gonna be at home with your mom? Blah. Fuck! It happened man.*

Acceptance is a powerful thing. It is not nihilism, submission, or giving up. It is a strange form of realistic optimism. Miguel got to a point where he accepted his vision loss was permanent, and he started to work on reorganizing and refocusing his life. He thought of his illness as a function of karma, a just punishment for sins of his past. This made MS easier to swallow in a way. The world was not unfair in his eyes. It was a bizarre form of accommodative coping.

He was treated by Dr. Ayala, one of my former mentors at USC during my fellowship training. She is a young and caring doctor who speaks fluent Spanish and is known in the MS community for her epidemiologic research on Latinos with MS. Miguel was first treated with Avonex©, an intramuscular ⊠-Interferon preparation given once weekly. Just as with Dr. Emily Spitz, this quickly turned into a nightmare. He hated needles so much he had not even finished his tattoos, and the medication made him feel drugged and hung over—and not in a desirable way. He started the medication in November 2010, but he shortly afterwards developed a relapse in February 2011 with incoordination of the right arm. This symptom improved over time, and he enrolled into a research study[5] where they would supplement Avonex© with an experimental hormone called ACTH (adrenocorticotrophic hormone). ACTH stimulates steroid production and causes numerous side effects such as weight gain and diabetes[6]. He tolerated the drug well, but a new MRI scan done in late April 2011 showed multiple active lesions, so he changed to Tysabri© in August of the same year. Since that time, he has been completely stable, and he even recovered well from his relapses in early 2011. His vision has remained unchanged over the past several years.

He made it through one of the most difficult years of his life marked by several relapses and the death of his grandfather from sepsis, but adjusting to life as a blind person has been no small task. Even the simple things we all take for granted are more difficult now. It is hard to shop because he cannot see price tags, so he has to pull out his phone camera app and zoom in on everything he wants to read. He used to use a specialized device called an Amigo©, but he prefers the discreetness of his phone. Unfortunately, zooming in on every tag and label is a laborious process. Reading is now challenging and sometimes more trouble than it is worth. There are audiobooks, but they are not quite the same to him. He used to love watching baseball, but he now describes it as "pointless" because he cannot follow the action. He can no longer play soccer because he has trouble following the ball, and it comes at him unexpectedly. Skateboarding is out of the question. He tried it once, and the left side of his body ended up purple. Living with low vision is a painstaking process which involves learning a thousand little tricks and compensatory strategies which slowly become instinctual.

By the end of the year, enough time had passed that he had already begun to move on with his life. He enrolled with the Braille Institute and was taking classes to learn braille along with learning other adaptive techniques. He picked up some sign language along the way. He developed ties to the Junior Blinds of America (JBA) and was set up with a mentor and counselor. Unfortunately, his visual rehab counselor was monotonic, uninspired, and uncaring, and he treated Miguel like a number in an overfilled caseload. Still, he had a great experience with the Braille Institute and JBA overall, learning not just skills but also perspective on life.

At the Braille Institute, you have those that are completely blind and were born that way and are happier than happiness itself. In my head, I was asking, "How can you be happy with all of this happening?" What else are you to be? Sad and shitty for the rest of your life or just happy because you woke up today? Let's go with happy. I met people with dreams looking for alternative methods to get where they wanted to go. That's awesome.

It is natural for people to feel a sense of kinship with those who share the same disability, and because of this, Miguel made many friends at the Braille Institute and at JBA. One of his friends named Christopher was a famous vandal—a street artist. He was far more visually impaired than Miguel because of complications of diabetes, but he used his artistic skills and other senses to make beautiful public murals with spray paint. Restaurants on Rodeo drive were paying him handsomely for his work. The two became close friends, and Chris was a tremendous inspiration. It was incredible to see someone excel in a craft despite such a significant disadvantage. Chris also had a stubborn hard-nosed attitude about his vision. He would try to do everything for himself, often refusing help when crossing the street to the point of endangering himself. This frame of mind proved infectious, and Miguel knew he had to find a way to be productive and get back into the work force.

It was HARD to find work because how do you tell a boss, "Hey; I'd love work for you." Give 'em a resume, speak your game, and say, "By the way, I'm kind of blind." What's he gonna say? "Ah, fugget about it. Get out of here."

Miguel is very insecure about his disability. His close friends know all the details, but he keeps it a secret from his casual acquaintances and old friends. When he goes to a restaurant, he will often pull the waitress or waiter aside to order privately because he cannot read the menu. He will simply ask for a specific item or for a recommendation. Occasionally, someone will call at him from a distance on the street, and he will holler back, feigning recognition. He has cut ties with many of his old friends associated with crime and drug use because he wants to live a different lifestyle. For a period, he was living off $900 a month from social security disability insurance (SSDI), the generosity of his parents, and old savings. He would collect recyclables and sell them for extra spending money when he had the chance. An elderly woman in his building paid him a small fee to do her laundry.

He applied for a job as a phone representative for the FBI, but he did not get the position. He eventually broke through and got a job working for the Knotts Berry Farm Hotel. Knotts Berry Farm is an amusement park in northern Orange County, and Miguel works there as a houseman, stripping rooms, cleaning linens, and dealing with general maintenance issues. It is exhausting work, and many people from JBA have come and gone, failing to manage the workload and the stress of the position. He works from 9:00 to 5:30 on the weekdays and 9:30 to 6:00 on the weekends. The schedule is for five days a week, but he is often looking for extra shifts during weekdays he has off. He has to take a minimum two-hour bus ride to work each way, so he wakes up at about 5:30am on weekdays and gets home at around 8:00pm. Sometimes, he will do overtime and get home at 11:30pm. He obviously would have preferred something more convenient, but he had no other options, so he jumped at the opportunity.

JBA arranged the program at Knotts Berry Farm Hotel, and it is in place to give opportunities to the visually impaired. Despite this, Miguel treats his work as he would any other job, viewing himself as skilled and capable of this specific task even though he has limitations. He approaches it with a certain professionalism, showing up on time and avoiding gossip and personal politics. If he has trouble reading the schedule, he will use the phone camera zoom trick. If he has trouble vacuuming because of stiffness in his right arm, he adjusts his technique or uses his left arm. He uses his sense of touch to compensate for poor vision when inspecting the rooms. It has all become comfortable and familiar. He likes being active and on his feet, and he never views it as a grind. Luckily, aside from a moderate amount of fatigue and the occasional feeling of weakness in his limbs, he lacks many of the common subjective symptoms of MS. This is a blessing I cannot overstate because many people with MS could not maintain this type of schedule. His work environment suits his personality. Expectations are high, but there is a sense of camaraderie. The workers help each other and look out for each other. He regularly helps a woman in the laundry department who has far worse vision. Despite his busy lifestyle, he still volunteers for Food not Bombs from time-to-time when he has a random weekday off.

He has also found time to develop the romance he had been looking for since he was a teenager. He first met Amelia when he was still at ATC shortly after he developed optic neuritis. They met when Miguel was singing a Charles Manson song out loud, and Amelia started singing along with him as she was also a fan of

Manson's music. He was blind and toothless from the bike accident, but they still hit it off.

I chummed her I guess. We were two weirdos at ATC. She told me I taught her a lot, and I was like, "What do you mean?" She told me, "You taught me to have fun." Fun is free. It doesn't have to be luxurious. We would take walks or do little dummy things. I fell in love with her because I didn't need anything to have fun with this girl. I didn't need drugs. I didn't need booze. I didn't need to go out to eat. I didn't need anything. We'll just talk and have fun. Nothing could compare to her.

They were not serious at first, which is not surprising given everything Miguel was going through when he left ATC. They have become closer over time, and the more stable their lives have become, the more serious and committed their relationship has been. He does not feel that he has to act tough around her or put up a façade. He tells her everything including his medical problems and his dark past. They spend time doing simple things such as watching movies together even though he has trouble following the action. He keeps this a secret so she can enjoy herself.

Amelia is successful in her own right, and she works as a private assistant for a chiropractor. She is younger than Miguel, but she is mature and conservative in her lifestyle. Part of the reason for this is that she was diagnosed with cancer a few years into their relationship. She has undergone extensive chemotherapy and has experienced many complications including chronic anemia. This has left her tired, depressed, and listless. She has required blood transfusions and other interventions. The doctors are hopeful, but her prognosis remains uncertain, and the side effects of treatment have been taxing. He has helped her during the worst of times, bringing her food and doing chores for her after rounds of chemotherapy. Illness has a way of making people narrow their focus and take life more seriously.

Ill health has made Miguel more serious as well, and he has thought earnestly about starting a family. He is very protective of Amelia to the extent that he encourages her to eat healthy food, and he advises her on finances and other personal matters. An engagement ring adorns her finger, but they have no immediate plans for marriage as he wants to become more successful and independent before settling down. There is still a certain sense of Amerindian pride: he wants to be a breadwinner if he is to be a husband. He is making great strides in this direction, working hard, practicing thrift, and saving money. Dental prostheses have fixed his smile, and he feels much more confident now.

Recently, Miguel has been looking towards the future and thinking long term. JBA has provided him a great opportunity, but he would again like to go back to school. When he first worked with his visual rehab counselor, he was resentful of his emotionless and nonchalant attitude towards the job. Over time, he has come to understand how hard it is to be a good mentor, and the experience has inspired him to pursue a degree in psychology and to become a visual rehab counselor himself. Amelia is agreeable to the plan, and she makes enough money to support the two of them while he is in school with their minimalist lifestyle. The future looks bright, and he fantasizes about someday buying his mother a house, a goal his father could never achieve with rising property values in Los Angeles.

Miguel has not touched drugs since before the diagnosis, and he no longer drinks heavily. He even quit smoking cigarettes because of evidence that smoking correlates with a worse prognosis in people with the disease[7]. However, making up for mistakes of the past takes time, and he looks back with a certain degree of disgust. His outlook is an unusual combination of optimism and regret. His values have changed dramatically over the years, and his biggest regret is spending so much of his time doing something which is so meaningless to him now.

What productivity do you get out of just kicking it...just chillin' or whatever? You go sit somewhere in a room for a couple hours, and you're done. What is something productive you've done? What a waste of time. Garbage. Those I called friends weren't friends, and they never will be. That gets to me all the time. I'm not a dopehead anymore. I became a realist. Not that I can tell the future, but I believe if you are working hard, you will get whatever it is you want. I don't let people say "no," that you can't do things. Fail five times, and you're gonna get it the sixth.

Miguel certainly has many of the characteristics of resilience which we discussed in Chapter Three and which we saw in my other patients. He is fundamentally a calm and tempered person who is in control of his emotions. He was more prone to anger and impulsiveness in his youth, but this faded over time as he gained life experience. Now, he is the epitome of a realistic optimist. He accepts his blindness as a reality but is confident he can progress in life despite this disability. He is not putting his life on hold and waiting for a revolutionary medical treatment. As I said before, acceptance is a powerful thing we should not take for granted. If he were in denial, perhaps he would still be at home on the couch, waiting and wishing for a miracle. Instead, he made his own miracle.

Since he was a young child, he has embodied the principle of self-efficacy, a philosophy fostered by his hard-working parents and his humble environment. The same street mentality which got him into trouble in his youth serves him well as an adult trying to live with a disability. He also has a logical and pragmatic approach to problems. He makes decisions to achieve short-term goals based on information in the here and now. He does not expect everything to be perfect, and he is willing to make sacrifices. He also has a strong empathy towards others and a humanitarian mindset. This reflects in the way he cares for Amelia and in how he helps those in his community. His desire to do something meaningful for others is one thing that helped to rescue him from existential Hades when he first lost his vision.

The one thing he has struggled with is reaching out for help. He distanced himself from his parents in his youth when he should have sought their counsel and assistance. However, his experience with JBA and the Braille Institute have taught him the importance of interdependence, and he has become increasingly willing to look for ways to benefit from the kindness of others and the resources around him.

The reason I interviewed Miguel is that his background is so different from all the other people I came across. I am sure I have had many patients like him without knowing it, but doctors and patients rarely discuss these topics. Miguel teaches us we are not the same person throughout our lives. Although our early childhood experiences have a profound effect on our personality and character, we can change dramatically and build resilience over time. Although it would be ideal to anticipate all the tragedies we will face in life, the reality is that life forces us to be flexible and adaptive. The things we fear most will never come to fruition, and things we never imagined will push us to the limits of moxie and resourcefulness. He also teaches us the importance of morality and empathy in the development of resilience. If he had continued on the path of his youth, he would have gone nowhere in life. If you do not respect your own standards of conduct and treat other people well, it is nearly impossible to have the self-confidence and insight to solve your own problems. Furthermore, it is even harder to build the meaningful relationships and interdependence needed to solve life's most complex problems.

Over the years, Miguel has developed a balanced and comprehensive approach to problem solving. He has some of the type A grit that Dr. Spitz has. He has a piece of the unflappable nonchalance of Dr. Bhat. There is little bit of fire in the belly we saw with Sandra Orozco. He has a combination of these traits. He is hard-working and ambitious but also patient and relaxed. He is not a brilliant academician, but he is street-smart, flexible, and practical. He is a jack of all trades and an ace of none. He has his own unique brand of resilience, and I know he is destined to live out his dreams.

CHAPTER EIGHT REFERENCES

1. From the now defunct Food not Bombs website. Previously available at http://www.foodnotbombs.net/new_site/index.php. Accessed 12/2015

2. Duffy MA. Living with Low Vision. *American Foundation for the Blind.*

3. "MRI in multiple sclerosis: correlation with expanded disability status scale (EDSS)"; Frederik Barkhof; Multiple Sclerosis Journal; August 1, 1999

4. Zapata-Arriaza E, Díaz-Sánchez M. Clinico-radiological dissociation in multiple sclerosis: Future prospects. *World Journal of Neuroscience* 2013 August; Volume 3; No. 3.

5. Berkovich RR. Adrenocorticotropic hormone versus methylprednisolone added to interferon ⌧ in patients with multiple sclerosis experiencing breakthrough disease: a randomized, rater-blinded trial. *Ther Adv Neurol Disord* 2017 Jan; 10(1): 3–17.

6. Berkovich R, Agius MA. Mechanisms of action of ACTH in the management of relapsing forms of multiple sclerosis. *Ther Adv Neurol Disord* 2014 Mar;7(2):83-96.

7. Miguel A. Hernán MA et al. Cigarette smoking and the progression of multiple sclerosis. *Brain* 2005 June;Volume 128, Issue 6, 1:Pages 1461–1465.

CHAPTER 9:
MINDFULNESS

"You cannot stop the waves, but you can learn to surf"
—Jon Kabat-Zinn

WE HAVE ALL had days where we spend virtually one-hundred percent of our time doing something productive or goal-oriented. We are inundated by work, household chores, meal preparation, exercise, paying bills, childcare, and many other responsibilities. Often, very little time is left over to take a step back and bask in our present state to appreciate ourselves and our surroundings. We have all experienced days or even weeks like this. Our figurative emotional gas tank is empty, and we feel we are just barely making it through the day. We are essentially on autopilot, merely reacting to the world rather than interacting with it. When we find ourselves in this pattern, it is very difficult to be resilient because we have so little flexibility and emotional reserve. We are one unlucky break away from psychological disaster.

One process we can use to break free of this way of thinking is the practice of mindfulness. Mindfulness is a method of becoming attentive of the body, the mind, and internal and external stimuli. Jon Kabat-Zinn, one of its great proponents, defines mindfulness as "The awareness that arises from paying attention on purpose, in the present moment, nonjudgmentally"[1]. Mindfulness seeks to control two of the primary aspects of resilience: emotion regulation and impulse control. It has been practiced for thousands of years and originates from Buddhist philosophy and meditation[2]. It has become popularized by modern psychologists and used to treat various conditions. In this chapter, we will discuss the concept of mindfulness and the practice of mindfulness meditation along with the science behind it. We will also see a connection to some related concepts from Buddhist philosophy.

When life brings us conflict, we are either ruminating about the past or worrying about the future. These thoughts bring about negative feelings, and we let these feelings run our lives. To be happy, we must defeat or at least channel these thoughts. According to the Buddha, "If with a pure mind a person speaks or acts, happiness follows them like a never-departing shadow." To be mindful is to purify your mind by intentionally forcing yourself to focus on the present and to focus on objective reality rather than subjective feelings. This trains us to take control of and reorient our feelings. The ability is like a mental muscle, and to practice mindfulness is to exercise this muscle until it becomes easy and automatic to focus on the present. The goal is to develop a regular habit of mindfulness meditation and to systematically change your approach to yourself and to the world.

Try out for yourself a brief self-examination below which I derived from a meditation described in the book, *Mindfulness: An Eight-Week Plan for Finding Peace in a Frantic World* by Mark Williams and Danny Penman[3, page 4]:

Lean back and allow yourself to rest comfortably against your chair. Relax your legs and allow them to fall into a comfortable position. Allow your eyelids to become heavy, and observe as the room slowly darkens.

Draw your attention towards your breath. Notice how air flows in and out of your body, and notice your chest rising and falling. There is no need to change your natural breathing in any way.

If your mind wanders, gently but intentionally bring it back to your breath. If this happens many times or you find it difficult to focus on your breathing, know that this is part of the process.

You may feel your body and mind relax. You may feel uncomfortable or annoyed that you cannot maintain focus. Either way, just take notice without being self-critical. Just allow these feelings to be as they are.

After a few minutes, sit up straight and open your attention to the external world.

This is a simple example of a mindfulness exercise, but we can apply mindfulness to anything in the world. You can eat mindfully, slowly appreciating each texture and flavor. You can walk mindfully, noting the feeling of your feet on the ground, your heart beating, and the surrounding scenery. It is impossible to be mindful all the time, but by forming a regular meditation practice, we can help ourselves develop the habit. It is the equivalent of remembering to "stop and smell the roses" in all aspects of life.

Penman and Williams suggest various exercises and meditations. In the "body scan" meditation, you shift your attention to each body part deliberately, studying all the sensations you experience[3, page 97]. In "the chocolate meditation," you slowly eat a piece of chocolate, scrutinizing the texture, aroma, and the entire physical experience[3, page 55]. In the "mindful movement meditation," you stand up and make simple movements, intently monitoring every tingle, twitch, and shudder you feel[3, page 120]. These exercises may seem silly when you read them on a page, but if you put them into practice, the benefits become self-evident. You can apply the same mindset towards routine activities such as taking out the trash or brushing your teeth. While you are starting a meditation practice, try to write down the simple things in life you appreciate and the counterproductive habits you would like to break. Every week, you can focus on relinquishing an old habit of negative thinking.

When I was recovering from pneumonia in 2013 and could run for the first time, I appreciated running differently. I was feeling my breath draw in and out. I was aware of my feet touching the ground, and I was seeing the world move around me. Greenery appeared more beautiful, and I noticed shops in my neighborhood that I had overlooked for years. I was running on the same poorly maintained sidewalks and noisy streets that I had run on a hundred times, but it was an amazing feeling. It was a distinctly different experience than simply running to complete an obligation. I became mindful accidentally. The practice of mindfulness is to do this intentionally—to take in the routine and ordinary as if it were novel and extraordinary.

One problem with having a disease like MS is that the condition provides ample distractions on top of the usual stresses of daily life. You may have gnawing neuropathic pain constantly in the background of your mental activity. You may have an indescribable fatigue that makes even routine activities exhausting. You may have insecurities about your physical limitations or fears about the future. Because of this, it is even more important to take a scheduled break from life to ground yourself, release stress, focus on yourself, and focus on the present. People with a "type A" personality like Dr. Emily Spitz and Sandra Orozco would benefit from this tremendously.

The boon of mindfulness is not merely speculation. We have used it in the clinical setting to treat various psychiatric conditions such as depression, anxiety, and caregiver burnout[4-6]. As pioneered by Jon Kabat-Zinn, this has been called mindfulness-based stress reduction (MBSR), and its goal is to reduce rumination and self-critique. Mindfulness has been used in people with MS as well. In a study of twenty-four people with MS in Tehran, the twelve patients randomly selected to undergo a sixteen-hour MBSR and conscious yoga program had better energy, emotional well-being, and overall quality of life[7]. We think the benefits arise not just from improving psychological health but also by decentering the self and promoting of self-efficacy[8].

In patients with neurological diseases such as traumatic brain injury, stroke, and MS, mindfulness practice can ameliorate fatigue[9-11]. Worry and anxiety are mentally exhausting, and when these combine with the fatigue typically associated with MS, the combination is taxing. When you improve your ability to self-regulate and narrow your attention, you are more emotionally anchored, allowing your mind a moment of peace[12-13]. Thinking about everything happening in your life will make you mentally weary—just like a chess player will be exhausted by the end of a long tournament.

It would appear people with MS are more susceptible to this than the average person. In a study of MS patients performing a simple cognitive task called the single digit modality test, researchers performed functional MRI scans on both MS patients and control subjects. They discovered MS patients had greater activation in the basal ganglia, frontal lobes, and various other regions while doing the exact same thing as control subjects[14]. This suggests MS patients literally require more "brain power" to perform the same task, explaining why they may be more susceptible to mental fatigue.

Mindfulness can help with various other aspects of MS as well. Several studies suggest mindfulness has a benefit in treating chronic pain in MS and related conditions[15-22]. It has grade "A" evidence for treating chronic pain in the setting of neurorehabilitation based on an evidence-based review[23]. MBSR is useful in treating depression, anxiety, and general stress in people with MS[24]. Some evidence supports that mindfulness benefits physical function in MS. In a randomized trial with eight MS patients, the participants had six individual sessions to practice meditation and received various audio and video resources. The practice included a movement-based meditation similar to the "mindful movement meditation" described by Penman and Williams. At a three-month follow up, the treatment group had superior performance in a motor task where they had to stand on one leg and balance[25]. The effect may have been more due to exercise than any spiritual benefit, but the finding is still intriguing.

DR. KRISTIN NEFF

I have discussed mindfulness as a means to calm the mind and take a break from the world, but we can use it to confront conflict as well. Once you are in a state of relaxation and inner peace, you can begin to think about your problems in a more objective and emotionally modulated fashion. There is a balance we can find between emotional avoidance and emotional strangulation[26]. The long-term goal is not just to be mindful during meditation but to be more mindful in everyday life. In this way, we are more attentive to the world, and pleasant experiences are better appreciated. It also helps us to deal with unpleasant experiences because we face them with a more grounded approach and an inner well-being.

This well-being is often lacking in people because we are so hard on ourselves. By virtue of this, one principle that has become associated with a mindfulness practice is the concept of self-compassion. One psychologist, Dr. Kristin Neff, has championed self-compassion and has dedicated her career to the idea. She found it to be effective empirically when going through a divorce and trying to console an autistic child, and she has extensively researched what she knows intuitively. To understand Neff's ideas, try the following exercise[27]: imagine you have a very close friend who is going through a difficult time. Perhaps they have lost a loved one or have been diagnosed with a serious disease. Think about what you would say to them to comfort and encourage them. Think about not just what you would say but also your tone and your body language. Self-compassion is the idea that we should treat ourselves with the same warmth, care, and concern with which we treat other people, but we often fail to do this[28]. We are harshly self-judgmental and self-critical in ways we would never be towards other people. Indeed, Neff's research confirms this as people tend to be more compassionate towards others than they are to themselves.

Neff believes self-compassion has three components: self-kindness, common humanity, and mindfulness. Self-kindness is loving yourself and providing your own comfort when you experience pain, suffering, or difficulty. It is to be tolerant of your own flaws and inadequacies[29]. Common humanity is the understanding that suffering and challenges are part of the human condition, and setbacks should connect us to other people rather than isolate us.

Whether you are a first-time parent struggling through a sleepless night or a victim of MS, there are millions of others like you, and knowing this is a powerful thing. Mindfulness is the open, present, and non-judgmental state of the mind that allows us to be in tune with our emotions.

It is easy to understand self-compassion when we think about the opposites of these components[30]. Instead of self-kindness, there is self-judgment or self-criticism. Instead of common humanity, there is the feeling of isolation or the belief we are uniquely cursed. Instead of mindfulness, there is automated behavior and rumination about the past and future. Self-compassion is distinct from self-esteem. Self-esteem often derives from achievements and comparisons to other people. It is the sense of superiority or at least adequacy in your peer group. Self-compassion is different because it is self-love that comes from within and is not dependent on accomplishments or ascendancy. We all have high self-esteem when we're productive and successful, but it is often a fair-weather friend that deserts us when tragedy befalls us. If my self-worth depends on being successful, healthy, and loved by others, what happens to me when I lose my job, become ill, or go through a breakup? Self-compassion provides a stable sense of self-worth. It is self-esteem without a context or basis. It is analogous to what humanistic psychologist Carl Rogers calls "unconditional positive regard"[31].

To have self-compassion is to forgive yourself[32]. Counterintuitively, this allows you to accept responsibility for mistakes and shortcomings rather than making excuses or avoiding confrontation. It is not the same as self-delusion or narcissism because when you forgive yourself for faults and misdeeds, it is easier to accept them. On the other hand, if you are brutally self-critical, it is much harder to recognize your mistakes, and you are more likely to convince yourself that you have done no wrong and the blame lies elsewhere. If you will admit errors, you are more likely to look for ways to improve, and you are more likely to apologize to others when necessary.

Neff's research suggests self-compassion significantly affects psychological health, resilience, and happiness. Scales of self-compassion correlate with some markers associated with resilience as described by Reivich and Shatte including self-efficacy and optimism[33]. People who have more self-compassion are more socially connected and have greater overall life satisfaction[34]. Self-compassion helps to foster adaptation and optimism in people with MS and other diseases[35].

There are various exercises described by Neff and others geared towards developing self-compassion. One of the primary techniques is to adapt mindfulness to incorporate this principle. Instead of meditating about your breath, your body, or inanimate objects, you would meditate about your own suffering and attempt to invoke self-compassion. This is a more active and confrontational process, and it goes beyond simple distraction and relaxation. You can incorporate self-talk and therapeutic touch into your meditations. It may seem awkward, but think of it as an exaggerated mental exercise to sharpen the mind just as you might make an exaggerated physical movement to train a muscle. As an example, try the following meditation which combines the body and breath meditation with a self-compassion exercise:

Lie down in a comfortable place such as a couch or a bed.

Relax your body, and take a moment to clear your mind. Close your eyes.

Allow your attention to move to your breath, and note your chest rising and falling. Listen to the subtle sounds that you make while breathing that often go unnoticed.

After a while, move your attention to your abdomen. Perceive any sensations in this area, whatever they may be. If you notice nothing, just focus on this area of your body.

Next, move your attention down to your hips. Then, slowly move down to your thighs, your legs, and your feet. Observe any sensations in your skin or in your muscles. Monitor any tingling, muscle tightness, warmth, or coldness you may feel.

Now, shift your attention back to your breathing and again study the inflow and outflow of your breath.

Slowly move your focus up to your shoulders and then to your neck. Realize any sensations you have in this area.

Finally, allow your mind's eye to feel the sensations in your head.

Draw from your mind a recent event or concern that has caused you distress. It could relate to your work or your personal life. Whatever it may be, allow yourself to relive this burden briefly. Become conscious of how this thought troubles and distresses you. Think about how it causes you pain and suffering. Think about how it causes you to worry, ruminate, and become distracted.

Now, become your own counselor, and give yourself encouragement and support. Tell yourself that you are sorry that this thought causes you discomfort. Remind yourself that hardship is not unique to you; we all share it. It is part of our life story, and it is part of what makes each individual special. Use the words that feel most appropriate to the specific circumstance.

Take your hands, and use them to comfort yourself with the power of touch. Massage the tense muscles in your arms, back, and shoulders. Rub your chest and stomach gently. Touch your body in a way that makes you feel relaxed and comforted.

When you are done, slowly open your eyes and allow yourself to take in the room.

Hopefully, doing this meditation will help you cast your problems in an optimistic light, and you will face them with greater confidence and tranquility. Some other recommended techniques include writing and journaling. If you are ruminating about a negative aspect of your life or your personality, try writing a letter to yourself with encouraging words from the perspective of a close friend or mentor. Remind yourself about all of your positive qualities and about how everyone has setbacks and has to overcome difficulties in life. If you would like to improve something in your life, talk to yourself with optimistic encouragement rather than with self-criticism and degradation. When you catch yourself breaking this rule, think about the pain you have caused yourself and replace your thoughts with more positive ones. Try to imagine yourself as a small innocent child, and approach yourself with an appropriately caring and delicate tone. What you do consciously and deliberately eventually becomes subconscious and reflexive, and this is when you go from being a self-compassionate meditator to a self-compassionate person. To find more exercises and guided meditations recommended by Dr. Neff, go to http://self-compassion.org

I think it is also valuable to develop your compassion towards other people. Being sympathetic toward those who are like us or who share our problems is easy, but often, we have subtle biases against people who are dissimilar from us. If you are middle class, it is hard to relate to the very rich or the very poor. If you are healthy, it is hard to relate to the sick or vice versa. This is more subversive than it seems because it undermines our sense of common humanity and our ability to form relationships with others. To combat this, try the following exercise:

Think of someone you know. It could be someone you know well like a relative or your partner. It could be a coworker, acquaintance, or someone you have just met. Think about qualities this person has which you admire. Are they attractive, intelligent, responsible, or honest? Think of this person's greatest achievements. What have they done which truly impresses you? It could be a grand opus such as starting a successful business or a simple kind gesture like consoling a friend in need. Consider this person's amazing talents or the sacrifices they have made. Imagine how difficult and grueling it must have been to do what they have done. Even if you do not know this person well, try to use your imagination to fill in the details, and view them in a very positive light.

I will give a few examples from my own experience. My wife is a speech therapist, and I have always had tremendous respect for her profession. However, I never get to see her work with children first hand, so it is difficult to fully appreciate the craft. One time, she recorded a session with a young child for instructional purposes, and I had the opportunity to listen to it. She was so comforting and encouraging with the child. She was affable and calm while at the same time pressing him to use different sounds and make steady incremental progress. Using creative songs, props, and games to engage him, she was so smooth and efficient. When I reflect on this memory, I appreciate how much of an expert she is in this craft and how much time and effort she spent honing this ability. I could not perform as well if I trained for a thousand years.

Another thought I have is of my sister, Dr. Sky Ellen Beaber. She is a clinical psychologist and the author of the foreword to this book. One time in my youth, I was on a road trip with a friend, and we visited Sky in San Francisco. My friend was very depressed at the time to the extent he was seriously contemplating suicide. I had spoken with him for hours but had grown weary of it. As the three of us talked over drinks at a lounge, Sky became his impromptu counselor. She was inquisitive, professional, and genuinely empathetic. She delved deeply into his troubles with palpable curiosity and concern, and she really tried to make a difference in those few hours. My friend is now in remission, and although Sky cannot take all the credit, I believe she helped him through one of his darkest times. When I think back on it, I am incredibly impressed that she put so much effort into helping a man who was essentially a stranger to her. After talking to clients all day, I would think she would grow tired of counseling, but she has such a genuine passion for therapy that it just came naturally to her.

Let your mind wander about this exercise. Be very lenient in your judgment, and choose optimism over accuracy. When you think about it, the world is full of amazing people, each with their own unique gifts that we seldom appreciate. You should also direct this same exercise onto yourself. Think of your more admirable qualities and achievements. Set aside what you wish you could improve and focus on the areas in which you are fantastic and exceptional. Think about memories that fill your heart with pride. Pride is an essential emotion because according to the Buddha, "What we think, we become." If you think of yourself as having good qualities, these attributes will become accentuated.

TARA BRACH

I give quotes from the Buddha because mindfulness has always had a connection to Buddhist philosophy. Some American Buddhists have been amongst its strongest proponents, and they have added their own perspective and flavor to the practice. One such person is Tara Brach, a psychologist who teaches meditation and yoga in the United States and Europe[36]. She has studied the use of mindfulness in healing trauma and in eating disorders[37]. She recognizes people often suffer silently and create their own unhappiness. This phenomenon can be more significant than the actual real-life tragedies we experience. She describes this in the following way in one of her essays entitled *Accepting Absolutely Everything*:

> *Perhaps the biggest tragedy in our lives is that freedom is possible, yet we can pass our years trapped in the same old patterns. Entangled in the trance of unworthiness, we grow accustomed to caging ourselves in with self-judgment and anxiety, with restlessness and dissatisfaction*[38].

The solution is in the title of her essay: accepting absolutely everything. This is a "radical acceptance" of everything about ourselves and our lives. We must accept our inadequacies, our pain, and all the changes in life. It is analogous to what Mabel Katz calls one-hundred percent responsibility (Chapter Seven), but it focuses more on acceptance than responsibility. Brach describes this in detail in her book *Radical Acceptance: Embracing Your Life with the Heart of a Buddha*. She explains the common humanity described by Neff, that imperfection is natural and expected. When you accept yourself, you ultimately become freer because you are no longer limited by what you arbitrarily determine to be tolerable and unobjectionable.

The opposite of acceptance is figurative slavery. I remember a patient I saw as a medical student who was in her mid-eighties and was relatively healthy. However, her husband died of sudden cardiac death when she was sixty. She was devastated, having lost the love of her life and what she described as a perfect marriage. During every office visit, she would complain of her husband's death and become tearful. My mentor at the time was the patient's long-time family physician and said the pattern had gone on for years, and my mentor had spent most of each encounter consoling her. The patient had essentially spent the last twenty-five years of her life mourning her husband's death. She could never get over it. The death of a spouse is perhaps the most difficult thing to face in life, but many people lose a spouse and go on to live happy lives. The prerequisite to moving on is acceptance. If you cannot do this, the fantasy of your former life enslaves you, and you will mourn forever.

I could give a thousand similar examples. Everyone seems to think they are not good enough or that they do not fit in. They are afraid to speak their mind because they feel people will not accept them for who they really are. People dwell over slights against them, both real and imagined. Much of the field of plastic surgery involves treating patients who are insecure about trivial physical anomalies[39]. There are women who stand in front of the mirror for hours, concerned about a slight asymmetry of their breasts. Some men obsess over their physique or their hair loss. Radical acceptance is about accepting not just the small things but also the big things. Accept the physical appearance of your body. Accept the quirks of your personality. Accept the trauma of your past. Accept that you have a disease. This is not the same as complacency. You can accept and love your overweight body while starting a diet or exercise program. You can accept that you have MS while seeking aggressive treatments. Counterintuitively, acceptance increases rather than decreases the chances of successful intervention because you approach your problems with a calm and logical mind, open to change but not desperate for it.

A great example is former South African president Nelson Mandela who was imprisoned for conspiring against the corrupt South African government, and he was facing a life sentence[40]. After twenty-seven years, political pressures led to his release, and he became a legendary champion of human rights. What is most instructive about his story is his mentality while being imprisoned. Instead of harboring resentment towards his captors, he accepted his condition and understood that suffering and sacrifice were part of life and necessary to achieve his goals. Here is one of his famous quotes which reflects this sentiment:

Difficulties break some men but make others. No axe is sharp enough to cut the soul of a sinner who keeps on trying, one armed with the hope that will rise even in the end [41].

Instead of wallowing in despair, he spent his time in prison as productively as possible. He became an official representative of political prisoners[42]. He formed the "University of Robben Island" where prisoners would learn from each other and discuss different topics. He studied the African language Afrikaans and attempted to persuade people towards his political goals. He met with various politicians who visited him, and he inspired a political movement despite being imprisoned. None of this would have been possible if he were full of bitterness and despair. He had to accept his circumstances to move forward.

This is true no matter what you are dealing with in life. Dr. Emily Spitz could not be successful in her career without accepting some uncertainty about the future. Dr. James Bhat could not practice as a psychiatrist or enjoy time with his children if he did not accept his current disabilities. Sandra Orozco had to accept the loss of her career as a hospital administrator before moving on to her new life of political activism. Miguel Hernandez had to accept the loss of his vision before he could begin to achieve his goals. Radical acceptance was not merely helpful for my subjects; it was essential.

This acceptance is not innate; we can forge and develop it over time. One can do this with a modified form of mindfulness meditation. Brach recommends a style of meditation more in line with traditional Buddhist meditation but incorporating her unique ideas. She uses relaxing sounds and encouraging instructions. Ideally, you would dedicate yourself to a regular practice, preferably at the same time and place every day. The basic acronym is RAIN[43]:

R: Recognize what is happening
A: Allow life to be just as it is

I: Investigate with kindness

N: Non–identification or Nourish with self–compassion

The first two components (recognize what is happening and allow it to be as it is) are traditional components of mindfulness meditation. Pay attention to something as it exists naturally—be it your body, your movements, or your environment. The next two components are slightly different. To investigate with kindness is analogous to "paying attention to the present moment on purpose." The word "kindness" emphasizes you should do it in a gentle and open way. Non–identification means to allow ourselves to experience the meditation objectively, devoid of a personal identity. Awareness of the self is prerequisite to worry and rumination. We want to meditate in a way that makes the self temporarily irrelevant. Nourishing with self–compassion is the incorporation of Dr. Neff's self–love and care into the meditation. The result of all of this is to be attentive, tranquil, open, inquisitive, and kind to ourselves. To find out more information and for free guided meditations, go to www.tarabrach.com.

NOAH LEVINE

Another proponent of Buddhism–inspired mindfulness meditation is the American teacher and counselor Noah Levine. His interest in Buddhism and mindfulness comes from both formal experience and his unique background. Although his parents were practicing Buddhists and active meditators, he rejected the practice in his youth and fell into a path of crime and incarceration. Growing up in Santa Cruz, California during the seventies, he found himself a natural nonconformist and kept getting into trouble. He started smoking marijuana at age six[44], a level of precociousness which would put even Miguel Hernandez to shame. Problems with drug addiction grew as a teenager, and he had several run-ins with the law. When he was in juvenile hall at age seventeen, he thought to himself, "Maybe I will try Dad's hippie meditation bullshit"[45].

He initially believed things outside of him would make him happy—success, relationships, sobriety, and material things. But these things never gave him lasting satisfaction, and he realized the same thing that Mabel Katz realized: Happiness comes from within. He accidentally discovered the concept of one-hundred percent responsibility from Ho'oponopono. As the Buddha said, "Happiness is a choice, not a result." He found mindfulness worked for him, and he ended up pursuing a degree in psychology and a career in teaching mindfulness. He has written several books on the subject and now leads classes and retreats. Life taught him that if you conquer yourself, you can conquer the world. As he puts it, "Going against the internal stream of ignorance is way more rebellious than trying to start some sort of culture revolution"[46].

One principle of Buddhism is that suffering is the doorway to happiness. Adversity often inspires us to alter our method of thinking and to change our lives. For instance, the suffering experienced by Sandra Orozco led her to rekindle her religious practice and to search for new sources of engagement and meaning in life. Some amount of misfortune is intrinsic to the human condition which we must accept and prepare for, but much of suffering is unnecessary and self-inflicted. Our zealous pursuit of transient pleasure and our intense attachment to material things often causes more harm than good. The Buddha said "the root of suffering is attachment"[47]. Many of our decisions have the potential to lead to suffering. If we engage in romantic relationships, we risk getting hurt. If we pursue a career or start a business, we risk failure. Levine believes pursuit of things in life such as love, success, and money are not the enemy; it is our attitude towards these things which can become destructive. We must find a balance and develop a healthy attitude towards the things we desire.

Levine warns of the "hedonic treadmill" whereby we become accustomed to our changing standard of living. Just like a person walking on a treadmill, you will stay in the same place no matter how fast you go. When I was in college, I used to love eating at a cheap Indian restaurant called Naan & Curry. Since I left, I have eaten at various nicer Indian restaurants. When I returned to Berkeley, California to visit my alma mater, I ate at Naan & Curry for nostalgia. The food was terrible, and I was sorely disappointed, having remembered it so differently, and I wondered how I ever could have liked it. My taste buds had become poisoned by too much pampering.

The researchers Brickman and Campbell studied this phenomenon in the 1970s, and they proposed the idea of a hedonic set point. In one study, they interviewed twenty-two lottery winners and twenty-nine people who had become paraplegic in an accident[48]. Brickman and Campbell also interviewed a control group for comparison and asked all the subjects to speculate about their future happiness. They found that winning the lottery had no meaningful effect on happiness as rated by the participants. The paraplegics had a decrease in happiness compared to before the accident, but in a few years, they expected their level of happiness to return to baseline. The subjects also rated the pleasure caused by seven ordinary activities such as talking with a friend or hearing a funny joke, and both lottery winners and accident victims rated these activities as less enjoyable compared to controls. Here are the data below with happiness rated from zero to six:

Condition	Past	Present	Future	Mundane Pleasure
Lottery Winners	3.77	4.00	4.20	3.33
Controls	3.32	3.82	4.14	3.82
Paraplegics	4.41	2.96	4.32	3.48

Levine suggests we focus on increasing our baseline level of happiness rather than on manufacturing circumstances to raise it temporarily. We must think about what makes us happy and what we value in life. He stresses the importance of investigation in mindfulness. It is not about ignoring our thoughts or distracting ourselves from them. It is about understanding our thoughts and turning our mind into an ally. A large part of unhappiness is our attachment to experiences and circumstances which are fundamentally impermanent[49]. We can always lose everything and everyone we love. People with MS understand this more than anyone. We have to find a source of happiness that transcends these things. We also have to be willing to let go of things, and Levine calls this an "internal coup d'état"[50].

Levine uses traditional Buddhist mindfulness meditation but also incorporates elements of Buddhist philosophy into his teachings. He emphasizes the importance of knowing yourself and fostering a loving and forgiving attitude towards others. An inner change will naturally improve your confidence, resilience, and interactions with others, and this will lead to new opportunities in the world. He values modesty and simplicity, but there is a middle way between indulgence and extreme austerity[51, page 34]. Having desires is acceptable so long as you do not have excessive attachment to them. There is a balance in life between longing and acceptance, analogous to the balance between assimilative and accommodative coping discussed in Chapter Five. You do not want to be a workaholic or a slacker living in your parents' basement; virtue is in the middle. You also must seek to understand and confront challenges and suffering as part of life. The Buddha believed no one can escape the four main sufferings of life: birth, sickness, old age, and death. To expand on this is what Kristin Neff calls "common humanity."

Buddhism also stresses respecting the cultures of others and appreciating the broad diversity the world provides. The philosophy is egalitarian by nature as all people from all walks of life can seek truth and enlightenment. Many modern forms of Buddhism have dropped the cult of personality and have diminished the significance of the Buddha himself. There is also the principle of karma in Buddhism—the idea that positive actions beget good outcomes and negative actions beget bad outcomes. When we help others and perform charitable acts, we feel good about ourselves and develop inner peace and confidence while improving our reputation. This ancient wisdom is still practical today. Levine also talks about the importance of both acceptance and adapting to change.

He wanted to put his ideas into practice and to give back to his community, so he started a non-profit called Mind Body Awareness Project (MBAP) to teach mindfulness to incarcerated juveniles[52]. The group teaches mindfulness meditation and helps to foster positive values and an internal self-esteem. Many prisoners report they turned to crime due to feelings of insecurity and inadequacy, and only a small subset of criminals are openly antisocial and proud of their delinquent behavior[53]. Strangely, young people in juvenile detention have a lot in common with people with MS. They are under a tremendous amount of stress and external pressure. They face a stigma from society, and they struggle with indignities the rest of us would never experience. Volunteers in MBAP go into prisons to teach mindfulness and other emotional learning techniques. Check out www.mbaproject.org to learn more about the charity and to hear some incredible success stories.

Levine has also worked with recovering addicts, applying the principles of Buddhism and mindfulness to help alcoholics and people suffering from drug addiction. In a way, Buddhism is the antithesis of addiction because it teaches that attachment and desire are the central cause of suffering, and addiction is the most powerful form of attachment. One thing I appreciate about Levine is that he advocates a broad approach; mindfulness should be a way of life, not just something you do. These ideas are not just useful to specific groups such as addicts, delinquents, or those with mental illness; they can benefit all of us. The applications for mindfulness are endless, and many practitioners add a distinct twist for specific uses and groups of people. The popularity of the movement and the science behind it are growing.

THE SCIENCE OF MINDFULNESS

Increasingly, scientists have looked into the underlying neurophysiologic mechanisms of mindfulness. In an experiment by Italian researchers (Tomasino and Fabbro) [54], subjects entered an eight-week course to learn mindfulness meditation and underwent functional MRI scans. Functional MRI (fMRI) detects increased blood flow in activated areas of the brain during specific thoughts or activities. The study found that during meditation, subjects on average had increased activation of the right dorsolateral frontal cortex. This is a very complicated area of the brain which functions in cognitive processing, working memory, and decision making[55]. The right dorsolateral prefrontal cortex specifically has been linked to behavioral inhibition[56]. Activation of this area may relate to taking control of one's behavior and response to the environment. This may be part of how one turns off the automated and pathological negative reactions to the outside world. The same study showed mindfulness decreases activation of the rostral prefrontal cortex, an area believed to relate to abstract thought and integration of multiple complicated thoughts[57]. Suppression of activity in this area may represent narrowed focus and the ignoring of extraneous information during meditation.

In a German fMRI study on mindfulness, Anselm Doll, et al. attempted to identify functional engrams of the brain and their relationship to meditation. They argue activation of the right dorsolateral frontal cortex mediates a "shift of attention back towards focus on the present experience"[58]. During meditation, this area of the brain demonstrates an interconnectedness to the right posterior parietal cortex which represents the "central executive network" (CEN). We think the CEN is a neural network related to redirection and refocusing of attention. Individuals in this study who had a high mindfulness score on multiple rating scales had higher functional connectivity of the CEN and other functional neuro–cognitive networks. The study also found that experienced meditators had greater connectivity compared to inexperienced meditators. This supports the idea that the mind is like a muscle which we can train and improve over time.

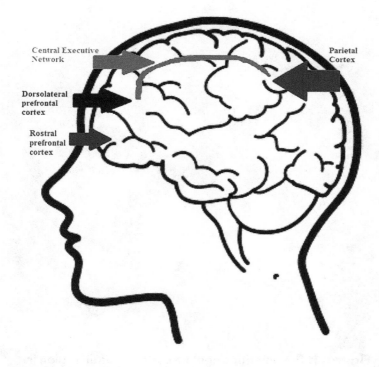

Figure 1: The central executive network (CEN) functionally connecting the dorsolateral prefrontal cortex and pari-

etal cortex. The CEN represents functional connectivity as found on fMRI studies, not an anatomical band of fibers.

The Germans also found a link between mindfulness and the connectivity of the anterior cingulate cortex and the CEN. We believe the anterior cingulate cortex functions in processing emotions and in inhibition[59]. This relates to the emotion regulation and impulse control mentioned by Reivich and Shatte as key components of resilience[60].

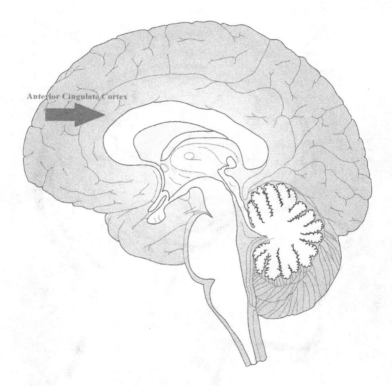

Figure 2: The anterior cingulate cortex: a brain region involved in processing emotion which functionally connects to the central executive network (CEN)

Anselm Doll's research presents an interesting finding regarding the default mode network (DMN) which is composed of the medial prefrontal cortex and the posterior cingulate cortex. Activation of these areas of the brain in concert is associated with mind wandering[58], and mindfulness inversely correlates with interconnectivity within the DMN. This corroborates the idea that meditation requires one to focus the mind and prevent mental wandering.

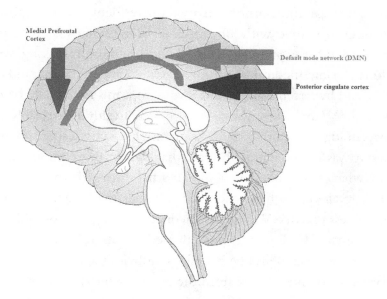

Figure 3: The Default mode network (DMN) functionally connecting the medial prefrontal cortex and the posterior cingulate cortex. The DMN here schematically shows functional connectivity but does not represent an anatomical band of nerve fibers.

In the book on mindfulness I mentioned earlier in the chapter (*Mindfulness: An Eight-Week Plan for Finding Peace in a Frantic World*), the authors Williams and Penman counsel us not to become discouraged if our minds wander[3]. This is because consciously refocusing the mind is part of the process. It is a useful exercise because it teaches us to develop the habit of mental fixation and to extend mindfulness into our everyday life. We are learning to shut down the DMN and to activate the CEN. The meditator is training the brain to focus on the here and now, and the neural pathways above describe the underlying physiological basis of this adaptation.

Because of these studies and others, the practice of mindfulness has gained traction in the medical community. Mindfulness decreases stress and burnout in medical residents[61] and improves wellbeing in people with amyotrophic lateral sclerosis[62]. It is also helpful in the treatment of anxiety and depression[63] along with various chronic medical conditions such as cancer, rheumatoid arthritis, and hypertension[64]. It improves symptoms in irritable bowel syndrome[65-67] and fibromyalgia[68, 69]. Physical health inextricably ties to psychological health, a truth humanity has known since ancient times. It was Hippocrates who said that "It's far more important to know what person has a disease than what disease the person has."

Encouraged by what we learned, my wife and I started our own mindfulness practice. We use the meditations suggested by Williams and Penman. We listen to guided meditations recorded by Tara Brach and Kristin Neff. The benefits are obvious and instantaneous. It forces us to take a break from the rigors of the day, to relax, and to gain some perspective. We spend time together after our children fall asleep instead of surfing the web or doing endless chores. We think about the Buddhist philosophy of Noah Levine and have learned more about Buddhism in general, trying to incorporate the principles which speak to us in our lives. If I am meditating and trying to be mindful, I am more likely to appreciate the little things in life. Seeing a follow-up patient who is doing well is more satisfying, and a long night covering stroke call is less exhausting.

The benefits of mindfulness are just as great for the healthy and privileged as for the sick and struggling. It is a way to prepare the mind to deal with conflicts and changes in the world. These problems may be things we are actively experiencing, but mindfulness is also a form of mental health prophylaxis. It makes us more resilient so when things inevitably go wrong, we are more prepared. Mindfulness is just one of many ways to achieve this, but the anecdotal and scientific evidence in its favor are quite significant. When you listen to people like Brach, Neff, and Levine, it is clear they are very resilient people. They are calm, centered, and judicious. They can take life as it comes, appreciating the whole picture, and acting rationally. Many of my patients have this characteristic, but perhaps none more so than Barbara Richardson, an incredible woman who is the subject of the next chapter.

CHAPTER NINE REFERENCES

1. Kabat-Zinn J. Wherever You Go, There You Are. *New York: Hyperion Publishing*, 1994.
2. Cigolla F, Brown D. A way of being: Bringing mindfulness into individual therapy. *Psychotherapy Research* 2011;21 (6): 709–721.
3. William M, Penman D. Mindfulness; an eight-week plan for finding peace in a frantic world. *Rodale*, 2011.
4. Shapiro SL, Kirk BW, Biegel GM. Teaching self-care to caregivers: Effects of mindfulness-based stress reduction on the mental health of therapists in training. *Training and Education in Professional Psychology* 2007 Jan;1 (2): 105–115.
5. Mindfulness-based cognitive therapy for depression (); Segal, Z., Williams, J., & Teasdale, J. (2009); New York, NY: Guilford Press, 2009;pp. 307–312
6. Germer CK, Neff KD. Self-Compassion in Clinical Practice. *Journal of Clinical Psychology* 2013 Jan;69 (8): 856–867.
7. Nejati S et al. The effect of group mindfulness-based stress reduction and conscious yoga program on quality of life and fatigue severity in patients with MS. *J Caring Sci* 2016 Dec;1;5(4): 325-335.
8. Bogosian A, Hughes A, Norton S, Silber E, Moss-Morris R. Potential treatment mechanisms in a mindfulness-based intervention for people with progressive multiple sclerosis. *Br J Health Psychol* 2016 Nov;21(4):859-880.
9. Ulrichsen KM, Kaufmann T, Dørum ES, Kolskår KK, Richard G, Alnæs D, Arneberg TJ, Westlye LT, Nordvik JE. Clinical Utility of Mindfulness Training in the Treatment of Fatigue After Stroke, Traumatic Brain Injury and Multiple Sclerosis: A Systematic Literature Review and Meta-analysis. *Front Psychol* 2016 Jun 23;7:912.

10. Wijenberg ML, Stapert SZ, Köhler S, Bol Y. Explaining fatigue in multiple sclerosis: cross-validation of a biopsychosocial model. *J Behav Med* 2016 Oct;39(5):815-22.
11. Tur C. Fatigue Management in Multiple Sclerosis. *Curr Treat Options Neurol* 2016 Jun;18(6):26; Tur C.
12. Immink MA. Fatigue in neurological disorders: a review of self-regulation and mindfulness-based interventions. *Fatigue* 2014;2202–218.
13. Valentine ER, Sweet PL. Meditation and attention: a comparison of the effects of concentrative and mindfulness meditation on sustained attention. *Mental Health Relig. Cult* 1999;2 59–70. 10.
14. DeLuca J, Genova HM, Hillary FG, Wylie G. Neural correlates of cognitive fatigue in multiple sclerosis using functional MRI. *J Neurol Sci* 2008 Jul 15; 270(1-2):28-39.
15. Grossman P, Niemann L, Schmidt S, Walach H. Mindfulness-based stress reduction and health benefits. A meta-analysis. *J. Psychosom. Res* 2004;57, 35–43.
16. Gardner-Nix J., Backman S., Barbati J., Grummitt J. Evaluating distance education of a mindfulness-based meditation programme for chronic pain management. *J. Telemed. Telecare* 2008;14, 88–92.
17. Teixeira ME. Meditation as an intervention for chronic pain: an integrative review. *Holist. Nurs. Pract* 2008;22, 225–234.
18. Rosenzweig S, Greeson JM, Reibel DK, Green JS, Jasser SA, Beasley D. Mindfulness-based stress reduction for chronic pain conditions: variation in treatment outcomes and role of home meditation practice. *J. Psychosom. Res* 2010;68, 29–36.
19. Chiesa A, Serretti A. Mindfulness-based interventions for chronic pain: a systematic review of the evidence. *J. Altern. Complement. Med* 2011;17, 83–93.
20. Veehof MM, Oskam MJ, Schreurs KM, Bohlmeijer ET. Acceptance-based interventions for the treatment of chronic

pain: a systematic review and meta–analysis. *Pain* 2011;152, 533–542.

21. Wong SY, Chan FW, Wong RL, Chu MC, Kitty Lam YY, Mercer SW, et al. Comparing the effectiveness of mindfulness-based stress reduction and multidisciplinary intervention programs for chronic pain: a randomized comparative trial. *Clin. J. Pain* 2011; 27, 724–734.

22. Lakhan SE, Schofield KL Mindfulness-based therapies in the treatment of somatization disorders: a systematic review and meta-analysis. *PLoS One* 2013 Aug 26;8(8):e71834.

23. Castelnuovo G, Giusti EM, et al. Psychological Treatments and Psychotherapies in the Neurorehabilitation of Pain: Evidences and Recommendations from the Italian Consensus Conference on Pain in Neurorehabilitation. *Front Psychol* 2016; 7: 115.

24. Kolahkaj B, Zargar F. Effect of Mindfulness-Based Stress Reduction on Anxiety, Depression and Stress in Women with Multiple Sclerosis. *Nurs Midwifery Stud* 2015 Dec;4(4):e29655.

25. Mills N, Allen J. Mindfulness of movement as a coping strategy in multiple sclerosis: a pilot study. *Gen Hosp Psychiatry* 2000;22(6):425–431.

26. Hayes AM, Feldman G. Clarifying the construct of mindfulness in the context of emotion regulation and the process of change in therapy. *Clinical Psychology: Science and Practice* 2004;11 (3).

27. Hayes AM, Feldman G. Clarifying the construct of mindfulness in the context of emotion regulation and the process of change in therapy. *Clinical Psychology: Science and Practice* 2004;11 (3).

28. Neff KD. The development and validation of a scale to measure self-compassion. *Self and Identity* 2003;2 (3): 223–250.

29. Neff KD. Development and validation of a scale to measure self-compassion. *Self and Identity* 2003;2, 223-250.
30. Neff K. Self-Compassion: An Alternative Conceptualization of a Healthy Attitude Toward Oneself. *Psychology Press* 2003;2: 85–101.
31. Carl RR. Client-centered Therapy: Its Current Practice, Implications and Theory. Boston: Houghton Mifflin, 1951.
32. Mickie F. Self-Forgiveness versus Excusing: The Roles of Remorse, Effort, and Acceptance of Responsibility. *Psychology Press* 2006;5:127.
33. Van Dam NT, Sheppard SC, Forsyth JP, Earleywine M. Self-compassion is a better predictor than mindfulness of symptom severity and quality of life in mixed anxiety and depression. *Journal of Anxiety Disorders* 2011;25:125.
34. Neff KD, Rude SS, Kirkpatrick K. An examination of self-compassion in relation to positive psychological functioning and personality traits. *Journal of Research in Personality* 2007;41 (4): 908–916.
35. Fournier M, De Ridder D, Bensing J. Optimism and adaptation to chronic disease: The role of optimism in relation to self-care options of type 1 diabetes mellitus, rheumatoid arthritis and multiple sclerosis. *British Journal of Health psychology* 2002 Nov;(Part 4):409-432.
36. *Tara Brach.* Kripalu Center for Yoga & Health. Retrieved November 28, 2015. Available at https://www.tarabrach.com/venue/kripalu-center-2/
37. Adelman K. What I've learned: Tara Brach. *Washingtonian Magazine* 2002, pp. 49–52
38. Brach T. Accepting absolutely everything. May 1, 2012. Available at https://www.tarabrach.com/accepting-absolutely-everything-2/
39. "Plastic and reconstructive surgery"; Maria Z; 2010; page 53

40. Eisenmann-Klein MZ. *Long Walk to Freedom Volume II: 1962–1994*. London: BBC AudioBooks and Time Warner Books Ltd ,2004.

41. Durando J. 15 of Nelson Mandela's best quotes. *USA today*, Dec 5, 2013.

42. Martin M. *Mandela: A Biography. New York: Public Affairs*. PublicAffair, 2010.

43. Brach T. FAQ for meditation. Available at https://www.tarabrach.com/faq-for-meditation2/. Accessed May 2016.

44. Sternberg D. From punk to Buddhist meditator. *Albuquerque Journal* May 23, 2004;Pg. F6.

45. LA Yoga. Teacher Profile: Noah Levine. Available at Layog-amagazine.com. Accessed 2012-04-19.

46. Levine N. *Dharma Punx*. HarperOne, 2004.

47. Bhikkhu Ñ, Bhikkhu B. *The Middle Length Discourses of the Buddha*. Wisdom Publications, 1995;page 868.

48. Brickman P, Coates D, Janoff-Bulman R. Lottery winners and accident victims: Is happiness relative? *Journal of Personality and Social Psychology* 1978;36 (8): 917–927.

49. Levine N. Against the Stream: A Buddhist Manual for Spiritual Revolutionaries. *HarperOne*, 2007.

50. Levine N. The Heart of the Revolution: The Buddha's Radical Teachings on Forgiveness, Compassion, and Kindness. HarperOne, 2011.

51. World Tribune Press. The Winning Life; an introduction to Buddhist practice. World Tribute Press, 2007.

52. The Mind Body Awareness Project. Available at Mbaproject.org. Accessed April 2016.

53. Schmideberg M. Psychological factors underlying criminal behavior. *Journal of Criminal law and criminology* 1947;volume 37, Issue 6.

54. Tomasino B, Fabbro F. Increases in the right dorsolateral prefrontal cortex and decreases the rostral prefrontal cortex

activation after-8 weeks of focused attention based mindfulness meditation. *Brain Cogn* 2015 Dec 22;102:46-54.

55. Nelson CA, Luciana M. Handbook of developmental cognitive neuroscience. *MIT Press*, 2001.

56. Shackman A, Mcmenamin BW, Maxwell JS, Greischar JL, Davidson RJ. Right Dorsolateral Prefrontal Cortical Activity and Behavioral Inhibition. *Psychological Science* 2009 April;20: 1500–1506.

57. Petrides M, Pandya DN. Efferent Association Pathways from the Rostral Prefrontal Cortex in the Macaque Monkey. *The Journal of Neuroscience* October 24, 2007;27(43):11573–11586.

58. Doll A, Hölzel BK, Boucard CC, Wohlschläger AM, Sorg C. Mindfulness is associated with intrinsic functional connectivity between default mode and salience networks. *Front Hum Neurosci* 2015; 9: 461.

59. Smith SM, Fox PT, Miller KL, Glahn DC, Fox PM, Mackay CE, Filippini N, Watkins KE, Toro R, Laird AR, Beckmann CF. Correspondence of the brain's functional architecture during activation and rest. *Proc Natl Acad Sci USA* 2009 Aug 4; 106(31):13040-5.

60. Reivich K, Shatte A. The resilience factor: Seven essential skills for overcoming life's inevitable obstacles. *New York: Broadway Books*, 2002.

61. Goldhagen BE, Kingsolver K, Stinnett SS, Rosdahl JA. Stress and burnout in residents: impact of mindfulness-based resilience training. *Adv Med Educ Pract* 2015 Aug 25;6:525-32.

62. Marconi A, Gragnano G, Lunetta C, Gatto R, Fabiani V, Tagliaferri A, Rossi G, Sansone V, Pagnini F. The experience of meditation for people with amyotrophic lateral sclerosis and their caregivers – a qualitative analysis. *Psychol Health Med* 2015 Nov 20:1-7.

63. Hofmann SG, Sawyer AT, Witt AA, Oh D. The effect of mindfulness-based therapy on anxiety and depression: A meta-analytic review. *J Consult Clin Psychol* 2010 Apr; 78(2):169-83.

64. Carlson LE. Mindfulness-based interventions for physical conditions: a narrative review evaluating levels of evidence. ISRN Psychiatry 2012 Nov 14;2012:651583.

65. Ljótsson B, Andréewitch S, Hedman E, Rück C, Andersson G, Lindefors N. Exposure and mindfulness based therapy for irritable bowel syndrome—an open pilot study. *Journal of Behavior Therapy and Experimental Psychiatry* 2010;41(3):185–190.

66. Kearney DJ, McDermott K, Martinez M, Simpson TL. Association of participation in a mindfulness programme with bowel symptoms, gastrointestinal symptom-specific anxiety and quality of life. *Alimentary Pharmacology and Therapeutics* 2011;34(3):363–373.

67. Ljotsson B, Andersson G, Andersson E, Hedman E, Lindfors P, Andreewitch S, et al. Acceptability, effectiveness, and cost-effectiveness of internet-based exposure treatment for irritable bowel syndrome in a clinical sample: a randomized controlled trial. *BMC Gastroenterology* 2011;12(11):p. 110.

68. Kaplan KH, Goldenberg DL, Galvin-Nadeau M. The impact of a meditation-based stress reduction program on fibromyalgia. *General Hospital Psychiatry* 1993;15(5):284–289.

69. Goldenberg DL, Kaplan KH, Nadeau MG, Brodeur C, Smith S, Schmid CH. A controlled study of a stress-reduction, cognitive-behavioral treatment program in fibromyalgia. *Journal of Musculoskeletal Pain* 1994;2(2):53–66.

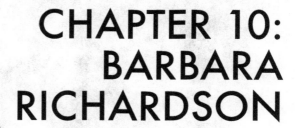

CHAPTER 10:
BARBARA
RICHARDSON

"Pray to me when you are in trouble!
I will deliver you"
—Psalm 50:15

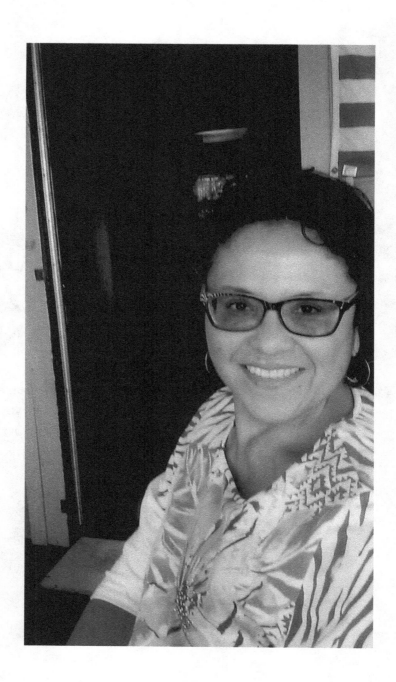

OUT OF ALL the people I interviewed, Barbara Richardson has by far the highest degree of physical impairment. She was born in 1961 and has had progressive MS since the 1990s. She has profound weakness of both legs along with her right arm, leaving only a dysmetric left arm to control her motorized scooter and to carry out daily tasks. Yet, her mind and voice are sharp, and she speaks with a transcendent wisdom few people possess. Exhibiting remarkable tranquility and optimism, she derives much of her support and strength from her large family and her Christian faith. She is active in her church and takes classes in Bible studies. She volunteers regularly as well, teaching English to those in need within her community. She is a leader in her family and helps others affected by MS. This is a story about how perspective, perseverance, and character are more powerful than any physical affliction.

Barbara's mother was born in Puerto Rico, and her father is a member of the Haliwa-Saponi Native American tribe of North Carolina. She has lived nearly her entire life in Los Angeles in an area south of Pasadena in the Monterey Hills neighborhood. Her mother had three children with another man many years before her parents married, so she has three older half siblings. They are so much older that she attended high school with her half niece. Barbara's parents had four children together, and they adopted Barbara's cousin who was five years old at the time. Hence, Barbara's generation has a total of eight people, and she was the middle child amongst the five younger children who grew up in their household. From oldest to youngest, there was her older sister, her cousin, Barbara herself, her brother, and her younger sister—four girls and one boy in all.

Her father was a strong man who worked as a lineman for the Department of Water and Power. He used to climb poles and hang transmission lines. Even now at eighty-seven years old, he is very active, and his age surprises most people who meet him. He was handy and hard-working, and he built their original childhood home with his own two hands. When Barbara was four, he had a major electrical accident at work, and he suffered severe burns over most of his body. He was taken to Good Samaritan Hospital, and the children could not visit at first because they were too young. For a short time after the accident, he was critically ill, and his life was in jeopardy. Luckily, he steadily improved, and they expected him to recover fully. They could finally visit on Easter, and she remembers his whole body covered in black eschars. He could barely find the strength to wave to his children, and she remembers looking with her sisters and saying, "He looks like a monster." When he finally came home, his eschars started to peel, and she would sit on his lap and peel scabs off of his skin. His ears were destroyed and permanently deformed. He had to have skin grafts, and he was out of work for an entire year. The finances were difficult for a while, but he went back to his usual job after the incident, and life went on as though the accident had never happened. They became used to his appearance, and when other children would ask, "What's wrong with your father?" she would say, "What do you mean what's wrong with my father?" Later, she learned to give an explanation.

Her mother grew up in Puerto Rico but later moved to New York where she met Barbara's father. In the 1940s during World War II, Barbara's mother worked in a weapons factory, and there is a newspaper article written about her as she was one of the top employees. For most of her life, she was a seamstress, working as a garment maker for different clothing companies and later specializing in quality control. She would go to factories and make sure everything was up to par. Later, she owned her own sewing factory, but the business was unsuccessful, and so it closed after only three years. She used to sew beautiful dresses, hats, shoes, and other accessories. When her husband was ill, she would use her sewing machine late into the night to sew little outfits. She would put them in small boxes, decorate them, and sell them to neighbors so the family could have an extra five dollars for dinner or for little luxuries. They never thought of themselves as being poor. Children are adaptable to their surroundings, and Barbara's parents never made them feel that they were missing anything. In fact, they were often mistaken for rich because they would wear their mother's clothing to school and were often the best-dressed amongst their classmates. Her mother was also a talented cook, and they ate well even on a budget.

There was a sharp contrast between the personalities of her two parents. Her father was an energetic and spontaneous man, always encouraging his children to be independent and leading them on new adventures. Her mother, on the other hand, was more of a worry wart, generally cautious and protective. She was a "hot headed Puerto Rican" according to Barbara, and she would get angry with her children when they would misbehave. Still, she was a very generous woman who would do anything for her children. She taught them about Christianity and respecting others. She was the rock of the family, a very attentive person and always picking up on subtle cues if you were having a bad day and needed reassurance or advice. Despite the large family, Barbara never felt forgotten or marginalized. In terms of their lifestyle and activities, her father got his way most of the time, and he raised them in a rugged, adventurous manner. She looks back on her childhood with fond memories and is close with her siblings to this day.

We lived in a house that's just a couple of blocks over the hill. I was probably about three or four, but I have such a vivid memory. There was a big loquat tree—the largest loquat tree in town. My father wanted to level it out, and the way he was taught to level it out was to turn the dirt under the tree into mud, so he had to let it soak. It was very soupy, and my dad invited us to go ahead and literally go swimming in the mud. When my mother came outside and saw us, she was not happy—yelling in a mixture of accented English and Spanish, "Hay dios mio Tom!

Look at the kids! They're all full of mud!" My father simply replied, "Oh, leave them alone; they're having fun!" I still remember being in mud up to my knees, and it was fun!

My father bought us an old retired racing horse. He had no idea how to buy a horse, and we called him Snaggle Tooth because he had no teeth. Also, his back was very sway. This is back in the 70s, and there was another horse ranch just over the hill here. So, people in the community got to know us real well because of our horse, Snaggle Tooth. It was getting loose all the time, and we would get phone calls. "You know your horse is over here." It was just exciting and fun. I remember when we were kids, our dad got us a monkey. We had it for like a week or something because my mother made him get rid of it. My brother, who was then about a year and a half, was holding up a banana in his hand, and the monkey, even though he was chained up, swung and grabbed the banana from him. My mother got upset, and so my father had to get rid of him.

Her father would frequently call the children into his pickup truck impetuously, and they would ride in the back (before this was illegal) off to an adventure. She loved the wind in her hair, the camaraderie, and the laughter. They would go to the beach at night to hunt for grunions, unusual small fish that lay eggs on shore. Bringing buckets and shovels to dig around in the sand, they would never find anything but always had a good time. They would roller skate, camp, and go on long road trips. When you have a large family, road trips and camping are the most economical form of vacationing.

I remember one year we were going on a road trip in our camper. It was one of those campers you put on the back of a pickup truck. It was in the summer, and it was very hot. My father told us as a signal if there was an emergency to jump up and down on the floor to get his attention. Banging the window didn't really help because there were two windows separating us from our parents—the rear truck window and the camper window. The ice box had a big block of ice in it, and it was starting to drip. There was also a box of Tide detergent, so without us realizing, the refrigerator is defrosting this chunk of ice, and it's wetting the bottom of this tide box. Because we were very hot, somebody moved the Tide box to open a window, but when they moved the box, all the soap got out because it had gotten wet. With all the air coming in from outside and soap all over, it felt like we were in a sandstorm. There's soap flying all over the place. It's getting in our eyes. We're screaming, and we're jumping up and down. Soap got into everything imaginable. It wasn't funny at the time because our eyes were burning with soap, but it's funny now that we think about it. As kids, we just had some good times when we were on the road.

Barbara has dozens of family stories to tell. They would go camping in the woods and tell each other legends of ghosts late at night. There is the story of the time her sister ran out of diapers for her newborn in a seedy part of town, so they used towels instead. There is the story of a bat getting into their motor home. They had many good times together, and even though it is so long ago, Barbara remembers it as though it were yesterday.

My dad used to collect old Ford Falcons, and there was one that needed a new starter. My sister and I wanted to go out. "Well," he says, "Here's the part," and he told us what to do. My sister and I put our coveralls on, and we got under the hood of the car, and we changed the starter. We were all excited when we turned the key and it started. Those are the kind of things that my dad taught us. He taught us how to get our hands dirty. He taught us how to screw and hammer a nail in a wall—that sort of thing. He taught us that sort of independence which I really appreciate.

At the time when Barbara was young in the late '60s, elementary school was divided into two semesters: A and B. When she was in third grade, Barbara was labeled gifted and skipped from 3a to 4a (skipping 3b), getting a half semester ahead and gaining access to a few special programs. As a result, she graduated high school in 1978 at age seventeen, but she feels the change hurt her social life. She was a shy kid with questionable self-esteem. When she went to middle school and had seven classes instead of one, it was hard for her to feel comfortable and to make friends. She remembers being in school and waiting impatiently for the bell to ring so she could walk home as quickly as possible. She never felt at ease in school and never performed particularly well academically—though she moved through the grades readily enough.

Her father saw how the dynamics of Los Angeles were changing, so he sent each child to Puerto Rico for a year of school. He also wanted his children to be fluent in Spanish. In 1972 at age eleven, it was Barbara's turn, and she stayed with her Aunt who was a school-teacher. She suffered from terrible homesickness, crying every night for the first month in Puerto Rico. However, it turned into a wonderful experience as she became fully bilingual and got to know her mother's side of family very well. By the end of the year, she was phoning her father and begging him to let her stay longer so that she could go to a cousin's wedding.

High school was easier for Barbara than junior high, and she made many friends and joined the pep squad. However, although her social life and overall confidence was improving, it was at this time she experienced her first medical problem. Over the years, she had developed scoliosis, and like many teenage girls, she was too insecure to wear the cumbersome and visible scoliosis brace. As a result, her spine curvature progressed to a staggering fifty-five de-grees. It was painful, inhibiting her growth, and was certain to cause long-term problems if untreated. She was actually home schooled for a year in the United States because her condition was so bad, and she eventually had to undergo an extensive spinal fusion sur-gery with Harrington rods at age fifteen. After a long recovery, she went back to school for the 11th and 12th grade. She also worked part time at the Social Security office while in high school.

After graduation, she worked with her mother for a year in the sewing factory, and she then went to Biola University, hoping to appease her father's vicarious ambitions and to earn a college degree. She was very independent as a young adult and was not afraid to try new things and travel to new places. When she was nineteen, she flew to the east coast with her younger sister to visit family. They rented a car and drove from New York down to North Carolina, stopping at various places along the way. They also flew to Puerto Rico together to visit their mother's family.

However, she did not enjoy the college experience and found she had a short attention span for the coursework. So, she dropped out and got a job working for the city of Los Angeles in 1981. Her career began with a position in the controller's office, and she later worked for the police department and the Department of Water and Power. She performed well and enjoyed her work, maintaining records, handling administrative duties, going to meetings, and doing secretarial tasks. During the LA riots, she remembers being afraid to leave work and had to discard her uniform and to exit discreetly at the end of each day. She has few regrets but retrospectively feels she gave up on college too easily.

She initially met her husband at a dance club, and they married in 1983 when Barbara was twenty-two. Shortly afterwards, they had a daughter. The relationship with her husband was often stressful and tumultuous as he is a flagrant alcoholic who would go through periods of sobriety and periods of drunkenness. Barbara tried to work everything out and provide a stable environment for her daughter, but there was only so much she could do. During periods of remission, he was a genuinely good husband and father, so she was intensely loyal to him. She also desperately wanted more children, but for a ten-year period, the couple tried and tried without success. She eventually went to see a specialist who diagnosed her with a bicornuate uterus, a condition in which the upper part of the uterus is divided into two sections. This leads to a cramped and anatomically abnormal uterus which can reduce fertility. The doctor said, "Well, I cannot really tell you that you cannot have children because you already have a child, but you have a bicornuate uterus, and that could be the reason you are not able to conceive." This troubled her greatly, but she was soon distracted by more urgent problems.

In 1990, she started to have intermittent numbness and tingling of the right side of her body. It did not worry her at first, but shortly afterwards, she developed blurry vision in her right eye, and an ophthalmologist diagnosed her with optic neuritis. They said her vision would improve in a few weeks, and it did. Strangely, no one mentioned MS at the time. During the same year, her husband got into a major accident while driving drunk and was facing criminal charges. She remembers trying to obtain an attorney, and while signing the paperwork, she realized her beautiful penmanship had become unrecognizable due to clumsiness of her hand. It was to where banks and court authorities would question her signature because it did not match her driver's license.

She first visited her family doctor to complain of these symptoms, and knowing her history of scoliosis, he took x-rays to make sure everything was in place. They were afraid to do MRI scans because of the magnetically susceptible Harrington rods in her back. As it turns out, two of the rods were broken, and this incidental finding proved a red herring that would delay her diagnosis of MS. Various theories were entertained, and she had a constant runny nose which led her to believe she could have a mysterious allergy. She eventually saw a neurologist who ordered an MRI of the brain, but this film was reportedly negative, so an explanation for her symptoms eluded her once again.

In the meantime, her husband's drunk-driving case proved indefensible, and he was sentenced to three years in prison, leaving the family devastated. Barbara found herself alone with her daughter, and she was suffering from an unusual and progressive illness.

As time went on, Barbara slowly worsened. Retrospectively, she believes she has had progressive MS since the early 1990s. Her walking began to decline subtly, and she developed knee problems. She saw various doctors who could not give her answers. One suggested she pursue knee surgery which she did, but her symptoms continued. She even sought the original surgeon who had performed her spinal fusion, and he was the first doctor to consider a diagnosis of MS, suggesting that she seek a second opinion from a neurologist in the United States. However, it was around this time when her husband was released from prison, and she set her own needs aside to bring her family together again.

One night in 1993 while working at the Parker Center Police department in downtown, she had a big surprise. She finished her shift at midnight, and on the way home, she was in a minor car accident. She had a few superficial wounds, and she went to the hospital for x-rays. Around the same time, she realized her period was late, and she took an over-the-counter pregnancy test which turned up positive. After a long and unsuccessful period of trying to conceive a second child, she was elated. In fact, her prayer for more children was answered in abundance, and she gave birth to three sons between 1993 and 1996, an unusual occurrence after having no luck for ten straight years. She finally had her tubes tied in 1996 after the birth of her fourth child.

Having children, however, did not stop the worsening of her condition. After the birth of her first son, she developed incontinence, and it was much more severe than typical postpartum dribbling. Her mobility continued to worsen, and she planned to get further testing, but subsequent pregnancies delayed her. Finally, after the birth of her third son, she underwent a new MRI, a spinal tap, and visual evoked potentials which confirmed the diagnosis of MS. Some images from her MRI scans in 2015 are below:

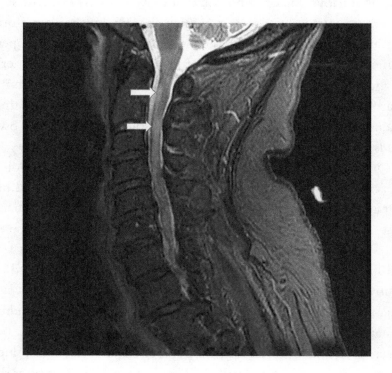

Figure 1: A sagittal T2 STIR MRI of the cervical spine showing extensive confluent MS lesions. Arrows mark a few of the lesions. She also has several herniated discs.

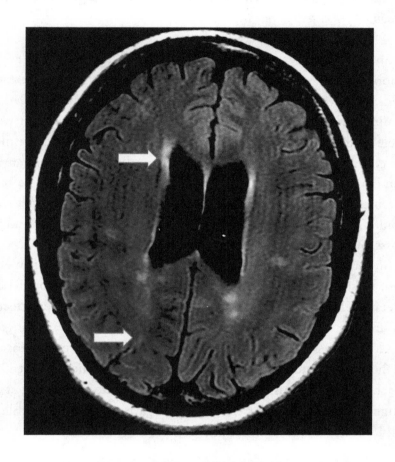

Figure 2: An axial T2 FLAIR image from an MRI scan showing MS plaques with relatively modest lesion burden relative to her overall disability. Arrows mark a few lesions.

When he confirmed the diagnosis of MS, I was actually relieved because finally there was a label to these symptoms I'm experiencing. I had a sense of relief because there was an answer. Someone is giving me a reason why I'm feeling this way.

She hardly knew what MS was before she developed the condition, but she was hopeful she was now on the right path to treatment. The MRI also found a small benign brain tumor called a meningioma, and she underwent local radiation therapy, but it was stable on follow-up scans and caused no problems. Around this time, she could still walk, though she was uncoordinated and constantly stumbling. She lives next to a large hillside, and even then, Barbara remembers having trouble chasing her young sons. She felt she would fall if she moved too quickly. These troubles became steadily worse over the years, though she had no distinct flares.

She started on Avonex©, the once weekly intramuscular injection. Despite trying for three months, her body just would not tolerate it. She would be doubled over in pain from the side effects, causing her to irritate her already aching back. She then changed to Copaxone©, a daily subcutaneous injection which was easier for her to tolerate. She took this for a while, but she did not like the shots, and she was clearly deteriorating despite the treatment at roughly the same rate. At this time, she gave up on standard allopathic treatments to look for alternatives.

I don't like needles to begin with, and back then, they didn't have the autoinjector. You had to do it by hand, and it was hard for me to reach certain areas. I think I just started reading things about natural ways to treat MS and became concerned about putting a lot of medicines into my body. I think it can be very confusing to someone because you read all these different stories of people that have just watched their nutrition and all that stuff versus traditional medicine.

She experimented with various diets and supplements. She would try a new supplement for three months, and if it did not have an obvious impact, she would drop it and move on to something else. Her persistence led her to Rosarito, Mexico to see Kurt Donsbach, a controversial alternative medicine practitioner[1]. He gave her monthly injections that contained vitamins and other substances. She would walk into the clinic with her cane, and within the hour, she would walk out unassisted. However, the effect seemed to be temporary, and the clinic soon got into legal trouble. Coretta Scott King, the wife of Martin Luther King, Jr., died of complications of ovarian cancer after consulting with Donsbach. The media attention led to Donsbach having his clinic closed by Mexican health officials. He later pled guilty to practicing medicine without a license in California[2].

No longer able to see Donsbach, Barbara continued looking for other options. At one point, she even enrolled in the famous low-carbohydrate diet clinic with Dr. Robert Atkins. She flew to New York and waited all day to see Dr. Atkins. She had several blood tests, spoke to his assistant, and received ample reading materials. Dr. Atkins himself spent only ten minutes with her and then rushed her out of the door. She tried the diet for a while, and she did lose some weight. However, she had headaches while on the diet, and she continued to have slow but continuous decline in mobility, so she eventually gave up on it.

She continued to work throughout the nineties despite her worsening condition. On top of her gradual MS progression, she had a flare with optic neuritis at one point. She also had a single nocturnal seizure where she woke up confused with a bloody self-bitten tongue. By 1997 when her sons were three, four, and five, she was walking with a cane. She was also having problems with her marriage as her husband continued to have alcoholic relapses. Her sixteen-year-old daughter was becoming strong-willed and would act out at times. By 1999, she decided that it was best to file for permanent disability rather than try to grind out a few more years of productivity. She was slowly becoming more disabled, and she wanted to spend some time with her children while she could still do most things. She left work, but she did not officially retire until January 2001.

I fell into a depression. It was noticeable just in the way my house looked and the way the kids were. Doing the basic things made me so overwhelmed. I went to the doctor—Dr. Spitzer, bless his heart. He saw me, and he was concerned when I went in there, and he gave me an antidepressant which I took for a short while. I was like, "I know I can pull myself out of this." This is just something that I need to face. And I did. I told myself, "No. You're better than this. This is just a temporary setback. You have too much around you that's important." I pulled myself out and got better without meds. I took it one day at a time through that dark period. I decided to be more proactive about where I was and to make do with what I could.

In the early 2000s, she was being treated at the Leslie P. Weiner Multiple Sclerosis Clinic at the University of Southern California. I did part of my fellowship training at the clinic, and I know Dr. Weiner well. He is a warm-hearted man who was a longtime chair of Neurology at USC. He had a legendary career and has a compassionate bedside manner truly worthy of admiration. At the time, he was conducting a randomized trial on a T-cell vaccine to treat MS, and Barbara participated in the study. She had to stay in the hospital for twenty-four hours every month to receive the vaccine. She had no side effects, and after completing the trial, she found out she had been receiving the real treatment rather than the placebo. They later stopped the trial as the vaccine was safe but not clearly effective[3].

Barbara continued to have gradually worsening mobility, and she started using a wheelchair in 2006. At first, she needed it intermittently for longer distances, but she became more and more dependent on it over time. Around this time, she had back pain related to her scoliosis, and she had surgery to remove her Harrington rods. In 2008, she separated from her husband and moved to South Carolina to live with one of her half-sisters. She lived there for three years just to put some distance between herself and her husband because the environment at home had become so dysfunctional.

When they finally got divorced, she lost health insurance because she had received it through his employment. Sadly, she did not qualify for Medicaid, and she had to part with her much-needed health care. She had been doing physical therapy to maintain strength in her legs, and when this stopped, it was not long until she could no longer drive. In May 2010, her leg gave out while she was driving, so she withdrew her driving privileges voluntarily, fearing she would cause harm to someone.

Later on, new oral MS therapies came onto the market. She went to a free clinic affiliated with Huntington Memorial Hospital serviced mostly by medical students and residents. In 2014, the Affordable Care Act went into effect, and she saw her previous neurologist who tried Aubagio©, but it caused terrible diarrhea. She had planned to try Gilenya©, but she did not go forth with it due to fear of side effects and lack of evidence of the drug's effectiveness in progressive MS[4]. She has effectively been without disease modifying therapy for the overwhelming majority of her MS history. Over the years, her leg weakness has progressed to the point of minimal movement. She has also developed gradual worsening of function in her right arm, and it is now to where it has very limited utility. She uses an electric power chair for mobility which she controls with her left arm.

Her overall health is not ideal either. She continues to have back pain and has significant spinal deformity from scoliosis. She sees a chiropractor regularly for adjustments, and finding a comfortable position in her scooter is difficult. Her vision is imperfect from old optic neuritis, and she often has difficulty seeing certain colors. She also has had a few general medical ailments. In 2015, she had pancreatitis which led to a long hospitalization. Because of the paralysis in her right arm, she overuses her left arm, and she has developed a shoulder cuff injury. She experiences an irritating neuropathic pain in her feet and has tried various medications. When the weather is hot, her symptoms worsen, and she suffers from disabling fatigue at times.

It feels like when you've been out in the ocean swimming and you're just making it back on shore. You just throw yourself on the shore, and you just can't move. Your body feels like you're carrying a fifty-pound weight, and you just can't do anything. You feel like you just worked out for two hours after not working out for years. It can be overwhelming.

Barbara works hard to maintain her body in optimal condition. She is not as stringent about nutrition as she once was, but she keeps a gluten-free diet and eats abundant vegetables. She uses an electric bike which moves her legs, helping to recirculate blood and prevent swelling and spasticity. Mid-day naps help with fatigue, and she wears a cooling vest that is stored in the freezer to combat hot weather. She is also creative in finding ways to adapt to her limitations. Using only her left hand, and she can still cook and put together a full meal. She keeps everything she needs in lower cabinets and even converted her dishwasher into another storage space for spices and other supplies. She will place a high friction fabric on her lap and use a cutting board to chop ingredients. Amazingly, she can peel a potato and do other things one-handed that would be impossible using typical methods. Her family built a custom ramp leading to her front door, and she will go outside with her scooter on her own to get a few items from a local market. She simply hangs grocery bags on the back of the scooter for the ride back.

Back when her children were young and she was still working, her husband's cousin stayed with the family and helped with the boys. After that, she was on her own. She tried to stay as active as possible now that she was no longer working. She would volunteer for her children's schools. She would find activities for her kids so they were not sitting in front of the television all day. She later volunteered at an organization called La Puerta ("The Door"), a community center affiliated with the Nazirim Church of Greenwood. She would teach English classes to those who wanted to learn. They had tutoring for children and adult classes in various subjects. They had a clothing bank for those in need, and they later expanded this to include donated furniture, small appliances, and other household necessities. The group started a public garden as well. A community formed around La Puerta, and they would have socials, potlucks, holiday celebrations, meetings, and other events.

The church has had a profound impact on Barbara's life. She was raised Southern Baptist and felt God in her life in all things from a young age. As a teenager, she accepted Christ. Despite her MS, she views the world and God as working with her rather than against her. Although many things have not gone her way, she feels she has experienced a thousand little miracles. She had four children despite a bicornuate uterus. Her youngest son was born with a ventricular septal defect (a congenital heart disorder) which resolved on its own without surgery. When she moved to South Carolina, she and her family found the perfect house immediately to meet all of her needs. When she needs help, it always seems to come. She will be alone at home and find herself unable to transfer from the toilet into her scooter, and someone will walk in the front door at exactly the right time.

Whether things were bad or good, it didn't matter. As I got older, my walk with Christ got close; it got better. I started reading more, and my relationship with Him changed. Too many things have happened in my life that I know were influenced by God. It was God. There was no other answer. So these other confirmations of Him in my life really bonded me closer to Him, and as I continue to grow, He's the center of my life. I'm living in His will, not my will, and that has really given me a lot of strength. The strength that comes from God has allowed me to continue going forward, learning to embrace anything that is going on in my life. This is a God who keeps His promises and is there when you need Him. When you're in a relationship with Christ, He teaches you how to embrace things and not whine about situations beyond your control.

She has become more serious about Christianity and Bible study over the years. When you are ill, it is natural to ask, "Why me?" She would sometimes think, "I could serve You and do Your will so much better if I could walk. I could do so much better if I could write." Now, she takes a broader perspective on her troubles, and she turns to scripture. As she says, she is living in God's will, not her will. This is the concept of letting go and trusting the universe as described by Mabel Katz and Ho'oponopono. Barbara reads devotions every morning, and a few of her favorite passages are below (New International Version).

John 3:16 For God so loved the world that He gave His one and only Son, that whoever believes in Him shall not perish but have eternal life.

2 Corinthians 12:9 But He said to me, "My grace is sufficient for You, for my power is made perfect in weakness." Therefore I will boast all the more gladly about my weaknesses, so that Christ's power may rest on me.

Isaiah 41:10 So do not fear, for I am with you; do not be dismayed, for I am your God. And I will strengthen you and help you; I will uphold you with my righteous right hand.

Her relationship with the church and La Puerta led her to pursue formal classes in Bible study which she began in 2017. These classes provide not just moral support and diversion but also a life philosophy. For instance, she takes the Corinthians quote above to mean she should accept her illness and be open about it. While many would feel shame for depending on other people, Barbara accepts it as part of who she is and feels little reservation about receiving the help of others. Luckily, she has a large and supportive family and can call her siblings and half-siblings when she needs assistance. She has a lifelong best friend who helps her as well. These people have been with her through thick and thin, and they supported her during her brief depression. They would come to her house and take care of her children so she could have a day off. They would take her to see doctors or simply get her out of the house.

Partly because of her religious conviction, Barbara lives her life spontaneously and opportunistically. She does not have any particular long-term plans, and she addresses issues as they come up. She is not free spirited or impetuous—just pragmatically hopeful. In this way, her mentality reminds me of Sandra Orozco, the political activist. When she signed up for the Bible classes, she did not even know if transportation was feasible. She just trusts that everything will work out. Her disability retirement provides a modest sum[5], and her long-term financial viability is tenuous, but she does not concern herself with this too much. She lives a simple but dignified lifestyle. She has everything she needs to be happy, and she has a deep-seated belief that everything will be okay.

Determined to keep herself busy, Barbara spends much of her time maintaining her home and doing activities with her family. She likes to go out to see movies or witness public events such as free concerts and youth baseball games. Her nephew is a professional boxer, and she watches his matches when she can. When you have a large family, there is always something going on. Her relatives, friends, and members of La Puerta meet for frequent prayer meetings. She does not have many other hobbies because most things she would like to do require two hands, though she can do some simple gardening in her yard. She can do basic trimming and can transplant a potted plant. If the weather permits, she likes to take her books outside and read in the open air.

Barbara is now back in Los Angeles, and she lives with her ex-husband and her two youngest sons. She is cordial with her ex-husband, and he spends about half of the year living with her and half the year in Mexico. He continues to have problems with alcohol, and when a relapse occurs, it throws everything into a figurative centrifuge. That being said, the family structure is more stable than it was in the past, and someone is usually around the house that can help her when she is in need. In 2009, her mother died of complications of heart failure at age eighty-seven. At age eighty-one, her father actually remarried. He is still very active with his new wife, spending time with the family and gardening. His wife sings and plays piano for the church, and she has been a welcome addition to the extended family.

Barbara has become involved with the MS community and frequents meetings organized by Familia Unida Living with MS (FULMS). Despite her preference for naturalistic treatments, she is open to learning about new scientific discoveries. When we first met, she questioned me assertively about many new therapies and appeared interested but skeptical. At her support group, Familia Unida ("United Family"), she met a woman with MS who uses a walker and is very depressed. They became friends over time and now speak almost daily. Despite being much more physically limited, Barbara is usually the one providing inspiration and encouragement. As in many other aspects of life, attitude is more important than situation.

The difference between Barbara and her friend with MS is not coincidental. She seems to do many things right and has many of the characteristics of resilience described by Reivich and Shatte in Chapter Three. She tries to control her emotions with prayer and meditation. In her youth, she would become easily frustrated with her health and her family, but she has adopted a philosophy of not worrying about things which she cannot control. If she becomes upset, she thinks about what is triggering this feeling and how she can change it. She is a woman of great insight and self-constraint. When someone wrongs her, she does not take it personally. When someone does her well, she is abundant in approbation. She uses the phrase, "It's gonna happen the way it's supposed to happen." There is a utilitarianism to this way of life. She knows when to push, when to pull, and how to read people, knowing exactly what to say just like her mother did.

She tries to be optimistic and to have a positive outlook, under-standing that people are drawn to those who see the glass as half-full rather than half-empty. She chooses to look at the good things happening in her life such as her children, her religious practice, and her involvement in La Puerta. Because of this, Barbara natu-rally attracts people, and they are happy to help her. It feels good to spend time with Barbara. It gives one a positive perception of disability, though she does not like to be called handicapped or disabled. She avoids criticism and complaint and was even hesitant to say a negative word about her husband when I pressed her. She reaches out to others deftly and has built a strong interdependence with her family and community. This has been difficult because, just like her father, she is independent by her very nature. She wants to do everything on her own that is not absolutely impossible.

She is empathetic to those who suffer from MS and to those in her community. It gives her great satisfaction to assist people in need and to volunteer. It gives her a reason to wake up in the morning and to put herself together. When you have a guiding reason to live, you do not have to worry about trivialities. In her view, everything is as it should be. She was not meant to work for the city. She was meant to stay home with her children when they were young. She was meant to volunteer at their schools and to raise them to have her values and character. She was meant to find a deeper faith and to spend time in her church. She was meant to connect with people with MS and with people in her community. Just as Martin Seligman describes, meaning is more important than pleasure.

Barbara's story shows us we cannot plan everything in life. When I think about my life, it is apparent to me how algorithmic and linear everything has been. I went to college, medical school, internship, residency, and fellowship. It was like clockwork with everything planned in advance. I established my career, got married, and had children. Throughout the process, it all seemed so arduous and uncertain, but looking back, everything worked out so perfectly. I am a very lucky man, but the reality of life is that you cannot depend on this linearity. There will be twists and turns. You must be flexible. You need to have multiple sources of self-confidence, and you have to be ready to find a new direction and a new purpose when things go haywire.

Barbara Richardson stayed just ahead of the curve while her MS symptoms were getting worse. The independence and hard work she learned from her father and the solid composure she learned from her mother helped her to cope. She is now like a wise owl in the forest, quiet and knowing. This is much more than an example of the hedonic treadmill. Barbara's ability to persevere has been an active process, the end result of decades of hard work, adaptation, transformation, and searching for new forms of meaning. Her accommodative coping style and religious faith did not arise out of thin air; they evolved over time. Barbara teaches us the importance of hard work, patience, and persistence. She shows us the benefit of a strong social network and how we can accept and adapt to virtually anything over time. Her story also demonstrates the tremendous power of religious conviction. No matter what I face in life, I will always remember her calm and determined countenance. She is truly an inspiration.

CHAPTER TEN REFERENCES

1. Tobar H, Richard Marosi R. Clinic That Treated Mrs. King Is Closed. *LA Times*, February 04, 2006
2. Perry T. San Diego-area man pleads guilty to 13 felony counts involving pushing bad medicine. *L.A. Now*, April 15, 2011.
3. Correale J, Lund B, McMillan M, Ko DY, McCarthy K, Weiner LP. T cell vaccination in secondary progressive multiple sclerosis. *J Neuroimmunol* 2000;107:130–9.
4. Lublin F et al. Oral fingolimod in primary progressive multiple sclerosis (INFORMS): a phase 3, randomised, double-blind, placebo-controlled trial. *Lancet* 2016 Mar 12;387(10023):1075-84.
5. Minutes of the Regular Meeting of the Board of Administration Los Angeles City Employees' Retirement System, 2002. Exact date and website concealed to protect her identity.

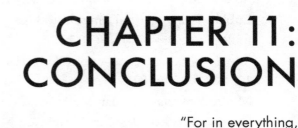

CHAPTER 11:
CONCLUSION

"For in everything,
it is no easy task to find the middle"
—Aristotle

O NE THING I learned in my research and experience is there is no single and uniform way to be resilient. The five people I interviewed are incredibly diverse. They are different both in their stories and their personalities. Miguel Hernandez and the psychiatrist James Bhat are very easy going and approachable. The neurologist Emily Spitz and the political activist Sandra Orozco have a mercurial fire in the belly. Barbara Richardson is somewhere in between. Both styles have advantages, and they all seem to make their personalities work for them.

They also have very different upbringings. Emily would call herself the daughter of hippies while James is the son of traditional Indian parents. Miguel and Barbara were both Latinos growing up in Los Angeles with blue-collar parents, but their childhoods could not have been more dissimilar. Barbara remembers jovial adventures while Miguel recalls disobedience and an early search for self-identity.

They all faced different forms of early adversity, and none of them had a pristine childhood. Two of them experienced serious medical problems in the family. Emily's father had a brachial plexus injury which left him with only one functioning arm, and Barbara's father had an extensive burn injury while handling electrical wire. Miguel had major academic and social conflicts along with frequent drug use from an early age. James had to deal with a fractured family, frequent moves, and an overbearing father. Sandra grew up in Compton and lived through the LA riots.

They also appear to use different principles of resilience which I discussed in this book. I wrote many of these chapters as though resilience is a quest that we must carry out in an explicit and organized fashion, but very few actually do this. For the people I interviewed, resilience came organically over time. Those who systematically change their lives through intentional philosophical paradigm shifts are few and far between. Even though James is a professionally trained psychiatrist, this probably has little to do with his resilience. Psychiatrists are experts in treating depression, but they have relatively high rates of suicide[1]. It is harder than we presume to change our personalities and psychological habits.

What one person regards as absolutely critical to their success is completely unimportant to another person. Indeed, key resilience factors are glaringly absent in some of my subjects. For instance, the significance of Christian faith for Sandra Orozco and Barbara Richardson is indubitable, but this was not a big factor for the other three. The workplace productivity for James, Miguel, and Emily has proven to be an invaluable source of self-confidence, but Barbara and Sandra gave this up yet continued to thrive. Philanthropy was a common theme, but the two physicians have little time for such endeavors outside of their work. Circumstances have made stable romantic relationships difficult for many of my subjects, so they search for other forms of social support. In the real world, no one can do everything perfectly. The failure of many self-help gurus lies in their belief that a few universal life strategies will work for all of us.

SIMILARITIES

Despite their differences, my subjects have some things in common. All five of them live relatively busy lives, and they have achieved what positive psychologist Martin Seligman would call engagement in life. As I discussed in Chapter Five, this is one of the three critical components of a happy life. When people with MS become more disabled, they often go through a very stressful period, trying to get disability benefits while learning to cope with daily life. The financial struggle is extreme, and I have had many patients go through multiple denials before receiving benefits. When they finally succeed, they feel a sense of relief, but depending on their situation, they may also face what I could call a crisis of engagement. Unless you are a parent with young children or have other significant obligations, giving up full time employment can leave you with too much free time. My experience is that unless you fill this free time with something, it can cause more listlessness than relaxation.

When I interact with Emily Spitz, she does not always come off as warm and amiable. She is more of a stoic character, but she is constantly doing something productive. When you are reading through journal articles or battling through a long night of stroke call, it is easy to forget about MS. Humans are unique in the animal kingdom in that we prefer to be busy rather than idle[2]. When they gave up their careers, Sandra and Barbara did well to look for ways to fill their time. For Barbara, it came naturally, and for Sandra, it was a long and painful battle, but they both made it happen.

Many would say that Barbara's life is boring. It is difficult for her to venture far from home, and her disability limits her to relatively few activities. However, she remains engaged by doing things many of us would find mundane. She takes pleasure in watering plants and going to the store. She is mindful in the mindful meditation sense even though she does not have a formal practice. If you have the right attitude, simple things can keep you distracted. If we feel the need to look for increasingly novel and exotic diversions, perhaps the problem is in our minds rather than in our lives.

Besides being engaged, my subjects also found a deeper sense of meaning in life advocated by the psychological schools of logotherapy and positive psychology. Emily did not pursue a stroke fellowship just to stay busy. She wants to be a part of something great. She wants to improve the quality of life of her patients and to advance the field of vascular neurology. She is willing to make sacrifices to achieve her goals, and this makes all the difference in the world. When she is facing difficulties in her career, she has a reason to persevere. She has a reason to stay active in her MS treatment. When she has a relapse, she has a reason to seek help and to facilitate her own recovery aggressively. She has a reason to learn to compensate for her symptoms whether they are apparent or invisible.

Sandra has also discovered a meaningful life. If she were not passionate about Southeast Los Angeles politics, getting up in the morning would be a wistful chore. But when you believe in your cause, you see every obstacle in your way as part of the path to success. Whether the obstacle is a corrupt system or your own body becomes irrelevant. Similarly, Miguel finds meaning in his relationship with his fiancée and in volunteering for Food not Bombs. James has found meaning in his psychiatry practice and in his family. Barbara has found meaning in Christianity and through La Puerta.

When I was a medical student, I used to volunteer at Salvation Army in a free clinic for the residents. The patients were so-called "beneficiaries" who were primarily recovering alcoholics and drug addicts looking to start a new life. We ran the clinic on Tuesday, and those nights were some of my fondest experiences in all of medical school. We would often run late and be tired the next day, but there was a special satisfaction the classroom and the hospital wards could not provide. There was something unique about helping the truly disenfranchised, and the patients were always incredibly humble and appreciative. I loved those guys. Also, there is something about the fact that we chose to be there. No one was making us do it. We were not there for a grade or even for clinical experience. We just wanted to be part of something.

That is one thing which distinguishes meaning from engagement. Meaning is the only thing which causes people to pursue endeavors voluntarily, enthusiastically, longitudinally, and in the face of major obstacles. One of my friends dropped out of medical school to become a professional poker player. He loved poker, and he could play for hours on end. His stratagems were elaborate and scientific, and he would recount hands with passion. He was quite successful and even paid his student loans with poker money, but he got burnt out after a few years and went back into medicine. Poker is simply not as meaningful as helping sick people.

SETBACKS

When I first spoke with my subjects, I knew instantly they had a tenacious and determined mindset, and I imagined that they must have been this way throughout their lives. It felt like a rigid and intrinsic trait. However, many of my subjects experienced significant setbacks and turmoil as adults. At some point in their lives, we could have described them as fragile and hypersensitive. When Miguel first developed vision loss, he was distraught and hopeless for a long period. After her MS diagnosis, Sandra was deeply depressed and suicidal, and she had no direction in life. Even the stalwart Emily Spitz was briefly anxious and emotional during her major relapse. If you met these people at the wrong time, you would have thought them to be decidedly inflexible and delicate. James and Barbara took their diagnosis and progression somewhat more calmly, but they too had their periods of despair. Of course, your judgment would have proven to be too rash as they all went on to be resilient over time.

The lesson here is the same thing I declared in Chapter Five: resilience is more of a process than a trait. It is complex and multifaceted yet tangible and malleable. You cannot buy it or wish it into existence. It is the birthright of years of struggle, learning, and personal development. We must have this in mind when we face our own setbacks in life. Even if you disappoint yourself today, you need not be the same person tomorrow. You can grow and change for the better. You can become the person you want to be over time if you are willing to be patient and make the necessary sacrifices. It often takes smokers thirty or more attempts to quit[3]. Normalcy and fragility are just as addictive as cigarettes, but just as a persistent smoker will eventually quit, we can all in time adapt to our circumstances.

MS AS A UNIQUE CHALLENGE TO RESILIENCE

In a way, having MS is more challenging and taxing on personal faculties than many other forms of conflict in life. In my research, I primarily found studies on resilience in response to uniphasic catastrophic events. These are things such as divorce, injury, war, terrorist attacks, and family tragedies. While these things are traumatic and surely test our resilience, MS causes different and more chronic problems. When a war veteran returns from imprisonment, he may have faced the depths of hell, but he will likely never return to dance with Lucifer. With MS, you are looking both through the windshield and the rear-view mirror. You have to think about what happened to you and what could happen to you. You imagine relapses, progression of disability, and all sorts of possibilities—both plausible and implausible. As I said, it is a naturally anxiety-provoking illness.

Because of this, people with MS need more than just the characteristics described by Reivich and Shatte. They need more than just a meaning in life advocated by Viktor Frankl. They need dynamic flexibility that allows them to face both the present and the future. This is a core feature that has allowed my subjects to thrive. When I look at Sandra Orozco now, she is significantly more disabled than when she was in the midst of neurovegetative depression. She is content and productive today because she has become more flexible. In her youth, she had defined herself as an able-bodied young medical professional, and when MS took this away from her, it was emotionally crushing. Now, she does not define herself so narrowly or allow herself to become too dependent on a specific form of success.

Barbara Richardson has done the same thing. As she declines over the years, she adapts not just her compensatory techniques but also her fundamental mindset. As she worsens, she establishes a new baseline of disability that she becomes accustomed to and accepts as reality. She changes her goals and expectations, focusing on what she can still do, and she actively looks for ways to enjoy life and find meaning. Even though her physical function is changing, she changes herself with the disease so she is always in equilibrium.

I call this process a dynamic equilibrium, a term used in the field of chemistry. A dynamic equilibrium occurs when two competing processes occur simultaneously to create a balanced but active state. For example, imagine a bottle of club soda. The fizz of the soda is caused by carbon dioxide dissolved in water. However, some of this gas is continuously escaping the water and entering the air within the bottle. An exactly equal amount of gas is dissolving back into the water because of the partial pressure of carbon dioxide in the air. Even though carbon dioxide is moving back and forth on the molecular level, the amount in each area remains fixed—in equilibrium. If I open the bottle and pour it into a larger sealed container, some carbon dioxide will escape to fill the larger air space. However, a new equilibrium will quickly form once the carbon dioxide gas pressure in the new container is sufficient.

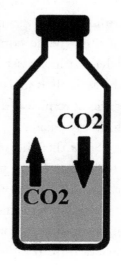

This is the form of dynamic flexibility needed for a chronic disease such as MS. You must be active yet accommodating. When the environment shifts, you too must shift to find a new equilibrium.

HAPPINESS

A prerequisite to being flexible is an overall sense of personal and life satisfaction. Much of the advice I give in this book about developing resilience is identical to the advice I would give about being happy. If you have a fundamental inner contentment, it is easier to develop the dynamic equilibrium needed to deal with the ebbs and flows of MS.

Happiness is an interesting thing. When I go to a restaurant with my wife, I am consistently more satisfied with the food and the service than she is. If she likes the food, I generally think it is outstanding. If she feels that the food is mediocre, I am thoroughly appeased. It seems absurd to me that anyone could be dissatisfied with the work of a professional chef, especially considering I am someone for whom a typical lunch consists of five pears and a can of tuna (while completing medical charts). It is almost as though I have a lower set point for satisfaction than she does. For other things such as social events and vacations, I am the one who is more difficult to please. If only I could have her wanderlust, and she could have my palate.

So is that the secret to happiness—just to accept the world as it is and to lower your expectations? It is not as simple as that because dissatisfaction drives action. If you do not have a least some amount of dissatisfaction and self-advocacy, it is difficult to have the motivation to improve your situation. I will tell you a story about inaction from my experience when I developed pneumonia while training as a fellow:

I was feeling ill with high fevers, so I left work early to go to the urgent care facility. The urgent care doctor did not know me even though I work a hundred yards away. He rushed the visit, and I did not mention I am a doctor because I did not want to make him feel uncomfortable or give the impression I expected special treatment.

He diagnosed me with pneumonia after a chest x-ray, and he gave me a prescription for an antibiotic. Even though I am a neurologist and not an internist, I immediately thought the choice of antibiotic was odd and different from what one would normally prescribe. I was not in the mood to cause a stir, and I generally trust allopathic medicine, so I did not mention it. Over the next few days, I became short of breath and ended up getting admitted to the intensive care unit. It turns out my pneumonia was caused by mycoplasma pneumoniae, a bacterium which has no cell wall. I had taken the antibiotic Augmentin© which works by inhibiting bacterial cell wall synthesis, and hence, it has no activity against mycoplasma pneumoniae. Generally, we treat community-acquired pneumonia with antibiotics that cover such "atypical" organisms. Would a different antibiotic have affected my disease course? Perhaps not, but the experience is engraved in my brain for eternity.

We must find a balance in life between enjoying our current state of affairs and striving to improve. This is true in almost everything in life—in our career, our friendships, and our romantic relationships. We all know people who complain about inconveniences or nit-pick about idiosyncrasies which we find trivial. We also know people with incredible apathy and lack of ambition. These people are rarely happy. Virtue is in the middle; you need enough happiness and optimism for psychological health but just enough malcontentment to keep moving forward. We should moderate this malcontentment and gear it towards things which are practically changeable.

IT TAKES A VILLAGE

In much of this book, I write about resilience entirely from the individual perspective. In a way, this approach is myopic because individual resilience is only one piece of the puzzle to managing a chronic illness such as MS. All five of my subjects have had significant help from their families and communities. Many of them had a childhood which fostered their personal character development, but perhaps more important than this is their social network in adulthood. Emily had the support of her mother and her husband during her major relapse. Without their help, it would have been impossible for her to care for herself. Miguel has the support of his parents along with a strong network of friends. If he were not so lucky as to have a place to stay and some words of encouragement, perhaps he would be on the streets living a life of crime. Barbara lives a dignified life with the help of her large family. Sandra maintains her independence mostly by capitalizing on the generosity of those around her. When I met her, a friend had dropped her off, and I dropped her off at her next destination. She just has a way of getting what she needs.

Social support ties closely with resilience and has many other benefits, both practical and emotional[4]. We know it correlates with resilience both in questionnaire scales[5] and in real life outcomes. A strong social network portends with various health benefits[6] and a lower risk of suicide[7]. Interacting with people meaningfully is a sign of a rich and fulfilling life, and the benefits of this fulfillment are innumerable and far-reaching. Conversely, social isolation is a known risk factor for various diseases including stroke, heart disease, and cancer[8]. People who are socially isolated are more often depressed[9], and people with MS and depression are especially socially isolated[10].

The benefits of a social network go far beyond financial security and a helping hand. It provides a source of pleasure in life when other channels disappear. It allows you to seek guidance during difficult times. It gives you an opportunity to support others and to form connections within a community. Miguel's involvement with Food not Bombs and Barbara's involvement with La Puerta fostered bonds of friendship and opportunities for altruism. This is the kind of social integration that makes people happier, more grounded, and more resilient.

RELIGION AND SPIRITUALITY

One special type of social support is that which comes from being part of a religious community. I knew about the importance of religion in resilience long before I ever became an expert In MS. This was patently obvious during my volunteer experience at Salvation Army. The beneficiaries came to the organization at one of the lowest points in their lives. I met convicts, people who had nearly died of an overdose, and men and women who had lost their careers, families, and friends in the throes of addiction. They had already dealt with the physical aspects of addiction such as withdrawal before they joined the community, but the beneficiaries needed much more than freedom from substances. They needed a new approach to life, and Christianity provided the support, discipline, and meaning to help guide them. I saw men and women with no high school education, nothing to their name, and a host of other problems develop a newfound confidence and purpose in life.

During the summer between my first and second year of medical school, we ran a high school equivalency test prep course for the beneficiaries. The goal was to help them become more qualified for jobs or for further education and training after leaving Salvation Army. Even though many of my students read at a fourth-grade level, they were enthusiastic and diligent. It was magical to see. Clearly, the religious nature of the organization has everything to do with its success. It gives the beneficiaries a reason to struggle for something better. For every challenge in life, there is a Bible passage or a wise pastor with an answer. It gives the staff a passionate career and a reason to get up in the morning, and this altruism inspired creation of the organization in the first place.

Hearing the stories of Sandra and Barbara affirms the importance of religion in developing resilience. Religion helps Barbara to find continued purpose and social support in the face of profound disability. Religion helped Sandra to bounce back from the depths of depression, and it allows her to go through life in a wheelchair with incredible passion and charisma. These two are the most seriously affected amongst those I interviewed, but they are in many ways the most content. Religion has provided them an identity, a sense of cohesion, a congregation, and a foundation of morals[11]. This quote from Sandra sums up the importance of religion in her life:

God has really been the force that I've needed in order to get through this, because without God, I just don't know if I would still be here. I probably would have died of depression sometime back feeling sorry for myself. It's so easy to give in.

There is scientific evidence for the psychological benefits of religion as well. In a study of 603 patients with kidney disease and/or type two diabetes, those who identified as religious had higher scores on a resilience scale[12]. Research also reports benefits of religion in spinal cord injury[13], cancer[14, 15], and AIDS[16]. Faith and gratefulness to God predict resilience in the poor[17]. In a study of U.S. military veterans, religion and spirituality correlated with a lower risk of posttraumatic stress disorder, depression, and alcoholism, and they associated with a greater sense of gratitude and purpose in life[18].

There are studies on religion and MS as well. In a 2004 project done at Portland State University, they examined fifty participants with MS to look for a connection between religion and spirituality and their ability to adjust to the illness[19]. They completed detailed questionnaires about their religious and spiritual beliefs along with a questionnaire designed to assess for psychosocial adjustment to

MS. Those with a greater sense of religious well-being had better psychosocial adjustment to the disease (R= 0.52 between the two metrics). Those with high religious well-being believe God is active in their lives and attends to their problems. These people had the same degree of uncertainty about their MS as those who were less religious, and they were equally likely to take immunomodulating drugs, but they were happier with their work and social relationships.

However, this does not necessarily mean that there is something unique about a specific religion or even religion in general. The same Portland State study showed that a sense of "existential well-being" had an even greater correlation with psychological adjustment (R=0.7) than religious well-being. Existential well-being in this study related to meaning and satisfaction in life outside of religion. Existential well-being and religious well-being correlated (R=0.75), suggesting that there are some underlying commonalities to well-being both within and outside of religion. The authors call the combination of these two traits "spiritual well-being," and they believe it is a marker of inherent coping ability, "spiritual drive," and meaning in life. These traits seemed to mitigate the psychological distress caused by the uncertainty of MS. Interestingly, some have reported that "extrinsic religion" (using religion as a practical tool to get personal and social benefits) is not as valuable in coping as "intrinsic religion" (being religious for its own sake)[20].

I believe a lot of techniques for developing resilience mimic the benefits of religion and spirituality. When positive psychologists encourage us to seek pleasure, engagement, and meaning, they could just as easily tell us to attend a lively religious service. The tenets of many religions foster the seven resilience factors described by Reivich and Shatte. Religious leaders encourage us to regulate our emotions and to control our impulses. Religious beliefs are intrinsically optimistic, especially when they involve an omnibenevolent God. Moral principles of religion teach us empathy and charity. A

Bible passage or Buddha quotation could justify many of the ideas I discuss.

Even a practice such as mindfulness meditation is in its nature a spiritual endeavor. It teaches us to change our mindset and to form a connection with our bodies and our surroundings that we would otherwise ignore. The result is a state of mind very similar to what we might achieve with prayer or chanting. Indeed, Buddhist philosophy directly inspired the guidance from many practitioners such as Noah Levine and Tara Brach. The principles of Ho'oponopono as advocated by Mabel Katz also have religious undertones. Ho'oponopono is a structured way of thinking and navigating through conflict in life. The concepts of self-responsibility, giving thanks, and having trust in the world are central to many religions. In fact, Ho'oponopono is primarily founded on a sense of faith in oneself and faith in the world.

Regardless of the specific tenets, methods, or metaphysics, it is impossible to deny the psychological benefits of religion and spirituality. Our ancestors had to face toils and deprivation which are rare today, and the religious community was a source of strength and stability. If these institutions did not build resilience, they would not have survived for millennia, and they would not continue to have such profound importance in the lives of so many today.

SHATTERED ASSUMPTIONS

Despite all these potential sources of strength, so many of my patients after first receiving a diagnosis of MS have uttered the same two words: *"Why me?"* The two words, actually, are pretty commonly heard following exposure to an unexpected traumatically stressful experience that is beyond one's ability to control, alter, or prevent. Before the experience, the person likely held a belief about life many of us hold. It is the belief that we control our destiny. That is, if we are good people who do the right thing and treat others well, good things are sure to come our way. Experts in the field of traumatic stress exposure have actually conducted research on core beliefs such as these[21] and have helped us to better understand how important they are to our emotional health and psychological well-being.

Few things alter these core basic beliefs. What will alter them, likely even shatter them, is exposure to traumatic life events. I have seen this happen with some of my MS patients. They now know something about life many of us remain unaware of. They now know that we have no control over each and every life experience that can come our way, some of which may be traumatically stressful.

But we can overcome shattered assumptions, and I have seen this happen firsthand with some of my patients. They confirm what researchers have found in the lives of those who eventually overcome traumatically stressful life experiences—that bad things beyond our ability to control or prevent can happen to us, but if we can rebound, we are better able to cope with future painful experiences[21, 22]. The suffering is not meaningless if it teaches us about ourselves, the world, and what we truly value or hope to achieve. It is not meaningless if it strengthens us. Without MS, Emily Spitz could not form the same personal connection with her patients. James Bhat would not have refined his views on psychological health. Sandra Orozco would just be another boring hospital administrator. Miguel Hernandez could still be an unmotivated addict. Barbara Richardson may have never developed her connection to Christ. Understanding this is a shift from a debilitating mindset to an enhancing and malleable mindset[23,] and if we adopt this, we are better prepared to live out the rest of our lives. Indeed, the purpose of life is not to live the life you are meant to live but to become the person you are meant to be.

A RETURN TO THE RS-11

In Chapter Three, we saw the RS-11 as a scientific measure of resilience, and I gave the survey to each of my subjects before our interview. They answered the eleven items below on a 1-7 scale ranging from "No, I disagree" to I agree completely[24]:

1. When I make plans, I follow through with them
2. I usually manage one way or another
3. Keeping interested in things is important to me
4. I feel that I can handle many things at one time
5. I am friends with myself
6. I am determined
7. I keep an interest in things
8. I can usually find something to laugh about
9. I can look at a situation in a number of ways
10. Sometimes, I make myself do things whether I want to or not
11. I have enough energy to do what I want to do

I totaled up the score to a value between seven and seventy-seven. Based on normative data from a German population, the average score on the RS-11 is 59.65. My patients had the following scores:

Dr. Emily Spitz: 68
Dr. James Bhat: 57
Miguel Hernandez: 74
Sandra Orozco: 77
Barbara Richardson: 61

Their average is 67.4 which is significantly greater than the German population (p =0.011) by nearly a standard deviation. The scores do not seem to correlate very well with degree of disability or productivity. Sandra Orozco responded "I agree strongly" to all the items, showing her tremendous self-confidence. James Bhat is the only one of the five to score lower than average, perhaps more due to modesty than a lack of resilience. If anything, I would regard James's ability to work despite his abnormal gait and voice as the most surprising thing I encountered. Resilience seems to come so naturally that he hardly has to think about it. Unlike Sandra and Miguel, he would not see himself as someone who has risen from the depths of hell.

Regardless of the scores, these men and women have reached heights very few people could achieve. They have overcome their individual challenges with creativity, plasticity, and grit. Despite MS, they live admirable and fulfilling lives, and they do so with incredible grace.

SUMMARY OF RESILIENCE SUGGESTIONS

Although my five subjects are all unique, they each teach us valuable lessons about resilience. Remember every day is a new beginning, and you can change and make yourself better, stronger, and more resilient. No single thing will help everyone, but I will leave you with this list of suggestions to help you cope with any conflict you may face in life:

Focus on your own happiness: As I wrote earlier, resilience correlates strongly with a sense of inner-contentment. Take Martin Seligman's advice, and search for pleasure, engagement, and meaning in life. Do things you enjoy, and spend time with people you love. Fill your life with activities, distractions, and important goals.

Try to think optimistically, and learn to look at the world through rose-colored glasses.

Form strong connections with other people: It is important to realize you simply cannot go it alone when you are facing a chronic illness or a major tragedy. Strengthen family ties and rekindle old friendships. Become involved in a community related to your interests, experiences, or religious beliefs.

Improve yourself: Search for ways to strive for personal progress and growth. This includes both practical abilities and psychological improvements related to resilience. What new skills or hobbies would you like to pursue? Which of the seven resilience factors from Reivich and Shatte can you enhance? The pursuit will be just as valuable as what you actually achieve. Remember to "broaden and build," turning bad luck into something beautiful.

Develop a logical approach to problems: Avoid excess emotion, particularly when it leads you down the path of despondence and self-criticism. Resist what Albert Ellis calls "self-downing," and train yourself to evaluate problems with an analytical mind. Break down large complicated problems into smaller and simpler ones. Make short-term goals and take immediate action.

Develop an accommodating style: If you face a dilemma with no solution, learn to accept that the world is imperfect. Remember that change and suffering are an important and expected part of life. It is something we all must experience, and in doing so, you are never alone. You are part of a shared experience of humanity with thousands, if not millions, of other people. Try to improve what you can change while accepting what you cannot change.

Seek religion or spirituality: If you have ties to a particular religion or philosophy, utilize this as a source of strength and support. Use the underlying principles as constant guidance, and become part of the religious community. If you are not inclined towards religion, search for other forms of spirituality or modes of inner peace. Develop a practice of mindful meditation or pursue alternate life philosophies such as Ho'oponopono.

Search for meaning in life: Think long and hard about your life's purpose. What is it you hope to achieve? What will be your legacy? What would make you most proud as you reflect on your life when you are on your death bed? In the background of your daily tasks and short-term pursuits, try to find an underlying meaning. Remember the wisdom of Viktor Frankl: "Suffering ceases to be suffering at the moment it finds a meaning"[25]. Conversely, if you do not have meaning in life, it does not matter whether you live or die.

Take care of yourself: In doing all of the above, do not neglect to care for the basic needs of your body and mind. Pay close attention to your lifestyle, diet, and exercise regimen. Get adequate sleep, and keep stress at a manageable level. Give yourself breaks in life, and fulfill your simple hedonistic desires from time to time. Nourish your body and spirit so that you will have the physical and cognitive resources to do all the little things that will make you resilient.

FINAL THOUGHTS

I hope that in reading the above stories and in learning about principles of resilience, you have found something to inspire you. Undoubtedly, you will someday find yourself in a situation where life seems unmanageable. You will be overwhelmed with stress, suffering, and apprehension, lamenting what you have lost and fearing for the future. It will be difficult to do, but try to remember to take a figurative step back. Look upon yourself objectively, and draw from all of your knowledge and experience that you have acquired over a lifetime.

Think to yourself, "What is it that will help me now? What resources can I use, and what strategies must I employ? Do I need to change my psyche by applying principles of psychology or by seeking formal therapy? Do I need to calm and refocus myself through meditation or other relaxation techniques? Do I need to search out help from others or be part of a community?"

My five subjects are in many ways extraordinary, but in other ways, they are just like you and me. Just as we all have tendencies towards despair and self-destruction, we also have the capability of resilience. When you think about the five stories, perhaps there will be one person you can identify with and seek to emulate. Perhaps you need a taste of Sandra Orozco's passion. In another scenario, you may need James Bhat's accommodative style. In yet a different situation, you may need the mental toughness of Emily Spitz. Always remember you have all these characteristics within you. You have demonstrated them at times, and you can call upon them again when you are in need. This is the amazing thing about us humans. No matter what happens, we have an incredible fighting spirit, and that is one thing that no one can ever take away from us.

CHAPTER ELEVEN REFERENCES

1. Merry N, Miller MD, Mcgowen KR. The Painful Truth: Physicians Are Not Invincible. *South Med J* 2000;93(10).
2. Raghunatan R. The need to be busy. *Psychology Today*, June 14, 2011
3. Chaiton M et al. Estimating the number of quit attempts it takes to quit smoking successfully in a longitudinal cohort of smokers. *BMJ Open* 2016;volume 6; issue 6.
4. Ozbay F et al. Social Support and Resilience to Stress. From Neurobiology to Clinical Practice. *Psychiatry (Edgmont)* 2007 May; 4(5): 35–40.
5. Weidong J, Guangyao L, Hua T, Ruohong C, Qian Y. Relationship between resilience and social support, coping style of children in middle school. *European Psychiatry* 2013;supplement1:Volume 28:Page 1.
6. Reblin M, Uchino BN. Social and Emotional Support and its Implication for Health. *Curr Opin Psychiatry* 2008 Mar; 21(2): 201–205.
7. Kleiman EM, Liu RT. Social support as a protective factor in suicide: findings from two nationally representative samples. *J Affect Disord* 2013 Sep 5;150(2):540-5.
8. Berkman LF. The role of social relations in health promotion. *Psychosom Med* 1995 May-Jun; 57(3):245-54.
9. Paykel ES. Life events, social support and depression. *Acta Psychiatr Scand Suppl* 1994; 377():50-8.
10. Mohr DC, Classen C, Barrera M Jr. The relationship between social support, depression and treatment for depression in people with multiple sclerosis. *Psychol Med* 2004 Apr; 34(3):533-4.
11. Ungar M. Does religion make children resilient? *Psychology today*, June 26, 2014

12. Estela J et al. Sociodemographic factors and health conditions associated with the resilience of people with chronic diseases: a cross sectional study. *Rev. Latino-Am. Enfermagem* 2016; 24: e2786.

13. Decker SD, Schulz R. Correlates of life satisfaction and depression in middle-aged and elderly spinal cord–injured persons. *American Journal of Occupational Therapy* 1985;39:740 –747.

14. Ell KO, Mantell JE, Hamovitch MB, Nishimoto RH. Social support, sense of control, and coping among patients with breast, lung, or colorectal cancer. *Journal of Psychosocial Oncology* 1989;7, 63– 89.

15. Colton SP, Levine EG, Fitzpatrick CM, Dodd, KH, Targ E. Exploring the relationships among spiritual well-being, quality of life, and psychosocial adjustment in women with breast cancer. *Psychooncology* 1999;8, 429 – 438.

16. Carson VB, Green H. Spiritual well-being: A predictor of hardiness in patients with acquired immunodeficiency syndrome. *Journal of Professional Nursing* 1992;8, 209 –220.

17. Bennett KM et al. Resilience amongst Older Colombians Living in Poverty: An Ecological Approach. *J Cross Cult Gerontol* 2016; 31(4): 385–407.

18. Sharma V, Marin DB, et al. Religion, spirituality, and mental health of U.S. military veterans: Results from the National Health and Resilience in Veterans Study. *J Affect Disord* 2017 Aug 1;217:197-204.

19. McNulty K, Livneh H, Wilson LM. Perceived Uncertainty, Spiritual Well-Being, and Psychosocial Adaptation in Individuals with Multiple Sclerosis. *Rehabilitation Psychology* 2004, Vol. 49, No. 2, 91–99.

20. Jenkins RA, Pargament KI. Religion and spirituality as resources for coping with cancer. *Journal of Psychosocial Oncology* 1995;13, 51–74.

21. Janoff–Bulman R. Shattered assumptions: Towards a new psychology of trauma. *New York, NY, US: Free Press*, 1992.

22. Katz M. On Playing a Poor Hand Well: Insights from the Lives of Those Who Have Overcome Childhood Risks and Adversities. W.W. Norton & Company, 1997.

23. Crum AJ, Akinola MA, Martin A, Fath S. The role of stress mindset in shaping cognitive, emotional, and psychological responses to challenging and threatening stress. *Anxiety, stress, & coping*, 2017

24. Rothe AVE, Zenger M, Lacruz ME, Emeny R, Baumert J, Haefner S, Ladwig KH. Validation and development of a shorter version of the resilience scale RS–11: results from the population–based KORA–age study. *MC Psychology* 2013, 1:25.

25. Frankl V. *Man's Search for Meaning*. Beacon Press, 1959.

APPENDICES

APPENDIX A

To give an example of the competitiveness encountered by Dr. James Bhat, here is a profile posted online by one of the recent matriculants to a BS/MD program[1]:

Class Rank: 1/590
Unweighted GPA: 4.0
Weighted GPA: 4.81

SAT: Math 780; Critical Reading 800; Writing 760 (2340 One Sitting)

APs : 9 (all Math and Science) completed by the time I applied to BS/MD programs, 4 more (Eng, Govt, Art, Psych) in senior year

Extracurricular: Scouting (Eagle rank), Field Hockey (Gold Medal - Nationals), Basketball (JV - Captain), Health Science Majors Program, Internship/Shadowing with Neurosurgeons, Medical Forums/camps, Public Service, NSHSS, National Honor Society, French Club, Student Ambassador, Youth Congress

Community Service: More than 600 hours combined from volunteer activities such as scouting (from feeding the homeless to constructing walkways at a local museum), hospital (Patient Pal), Hospice (Teen Mentor Program, Founder. Also helped get a $30K grant), American Cancer Society.

Research Experience: Some research under Biology Professor at a local university

APPENDIX B: THE CITY OF BELL SCANDAL

I edited this story from the original manuscript for brevity. It is an account of how local politicians abused their power to accumulate ridiculous salaries far in excess of what would be typical for a local administrator in a small city. The Bell scandal is a dizzying chronicle. Perhaps the main story is best described by the court of appeals decision:

> *A charter city is under the control of individuals who are looting the city's coffers for their own benefit*[2]

Some key players in the story are as follows:

Robert Rizzo: City of Bell Manager
Angela Spaccia: Assistant Chief Administrative Officer of the City of Bell, hired by Robert Rizzo
Randy Adams: City of Bell Chief of Police
Ruben Vives: A Los Angeles Times journalist who broke the story of the bell scandal

I'll start with the salaries. Rizzo received a base salary of $787,500 and a generous benefits package making his total compensation over $1,000,000 in value[2]. Needless to say, this level of compensation for an employee of a tiny city is absurd. The population of the city of Bell is only about 35,000, and I had never even heard of the city despite living in Los Angeles for most of my life until I learned about the scandal. Even Barack Obama only earned $400,000 annually while serving as President of the United States. Angela Spaccia had a base salary of $336,000. While other city employees were being laid off, Rizzo arranged his service credit to accrue at double the normal rate, allowing for double retirement benefits. He had 107 vacation days and thirty-six sick days out of only approximately 250 working days per year, and he could cash in much of this unused time for $360,000 on top of his base salary. Angela Spaccia pulled a similar trick, boosting her income by $175,000 in 2009. The city council did not approve these contracts, and he and Angela Spaccia went to great lengths to conceal their salaries. An e-mail to Randy Adams reads as follows: "We have crafted our agreements carefully so we do not draw attention to our pay"[3].

Randy Adams, the city of Bell Chief of police, received a base salary of $457,000 along with a favorable benefits package including lifetime health insurance for his dependents. Rizzo and Adams also had a prior agreement whereby Rizzo would support Adams' claim for medical disability upon his retirement from the city of Bell.

The excess spread to all the councilmembers. Oscar Hernandez, Teresa Jacobo, George Mirabal, Victor Bello, and George Cole all received $8,000 per month in compensation. These councilmembers were only part-time employees, and by law, a city a small as Bell could only pay councilmembers $400 per month[4]. The council absurdly passed an ordinance titled "limited compensation for members of the City Council" which actually increased their compensation. They justified their salaries by placing the councilmembers on a myriad of city agencies including the Community Redevelopment Agency, the Community Housing Authority, the Planning Commission, the Public Financing Authority, the Surplus Property Authority, and the Solid Waste and Recycling Authority[5]. That's quite an array of specializations for a group of people who worked part time and gained the position by receiving only a few hundred votes[6]. Again, Rizzo went to great lengths to conceal these salaries. He prepared a memorandum for the city clerk which fraudulently misstated the salaries of city employees. The memorandum stated that a Councilmember received $673 per month when they actually received $7,600 per month. Of note, even the $673 would be greater than the legally allowable $400 per month. The memorandum stated that Rizzo was paid $15,478 per month when he was paid well over $50,000 per month[2].

When asked to comment on their high salaries, Robert Rizzo and Angela Spaccia did not seem to be particularly apologetic.

If that's a number people choke on, maybe I'm in the wrong business. I could go into private business and make that money. This council has compensated me for the job I've done.—Robert Rizzo[5]

I would have to argue you get what you pay for. —Angela Spaccia[5]

While the Bell city officials were making out like bandits, the nearby City of Maywood was suffering. By attending Council meetings, Sandra found out that the City of Maywood had become insolvent. They failed to maintain the city insurance through the Joint Powers Insurance Authority (JPIA). The broad city insurance covered natural disasters, health insurance, and the pension for city employees. Part of the problem was incompetence because the Council failed to appoint a permanent city manager, a requirement for the insurance. However, the main problem was that they simply could not pay the premiums. Sandra herself went to the JPIA corporate office to plead on behalf of the city, but it was all for naught. The city of Maywood had to lay off 100 employees, and they lost their local police department which had been present in Maywood since 1923. Maywood had to raise city taxes[7], and financial problems have been present ever since 2010. Maywood was the only city to lose JPIA insurance out of over 200 cities that the company insures

Sandra believes that the Bell scandal directly relates to the downfall of the city of Maywood. In February 2010, Spaccia came to Maywood to serve as acting city manager for Maywood. Sandra became familiar with Spaccia because she attended city council meetings regularly, and Sandra became somewhat suspicious that Spaccia could be a mole. When Spaccia moved from Bell to Maywood, she took one of her secretaries with her. Sandra learned from an informant that this secretary earned an outrageous salary for part time work. Sandra met with other Maywood residents and one of her friends, Ruben Vives, a well-known journalist for the LA times. They knew each other because Vives would regularly attend city council meetings.

The group met at a Denny's at the corner of Atlantic and Slauson, and that's when it all started. They talked about the disbanding of the Maywood Police department and the layoffs of city employees. They talked about the pending contracts of city services with the city of Bell. They knew something was wrong.

Go across the tracks. Something is coming over here. There's something wrong.

Vives and his colleague Jeff Gottlieb then contacted the district attorney's office to ask about Maywood and accidentally learned about an investigation into the city of Bell council's high salaries. Ruben and the LA times were able to get information about all the city of Bell administrative salaries via the California Public Records Act. When the story went to press, the public outrage was palpable.

Bell residents took to the streets with picket signs, demanding justice and the resignation of the city councilmembers. There was a buzz of renewed political fervor within the community. The passion for justice was so intense that the journalists Vives and Gottlieb were receiving high fives and free meals from locals. Sandra Orozco spoke at a council meeting, and she lashed out assertively against one of the councilmembers, Theresa Jacobo.

I'll never forget the day that I went up there. I was in my walker. I went up to the podium. There were tons of people. The media was there.

"Theresa Jacobo: you're a damned liar. You need to go to jail, and you need to go to jail right now." And so I prophesied. Within ten hours, that's what the FBI did: they took all of them.

In the criminal trials, the evidence was overwhelming, particularly the e-mail exchanges between the defendants. Reading the news stories and court decisions would turn the most naïve idealist into a hardened cynic. In an e-mail to Spaccia, Randy Adams wrote, "I am looking forward to seeing you and taking all of Bell's money?!" Spaccia replied, "LOL...well you can take your share of the pie...just like us!!! We will all get fat together...Bob has an expression he likes to use on occasion...Pigs get Fat...Hogs get slaughtered!!! So long as we're not Hogs...all is well!![8]"

They sentenced Angela Spaccia to eleven years, eight months[8]. Robert Rizzo got twelve years in state prison and had to pay $9,000,000 in restitution[9]. Most of the council members also went to jail including the woman personally named by Sandra, Theresa Jacobo, who served two years in prison[10, 11]. Ruben Vives won the Pulitzer Prize and the Selden Ring Award for Investigative Reporting. Sandra Orozco became well known within Maywood politics.

APPENDIX C: RS-11 SURVEY RESULTS

These are the results of the RS-11 survey used by Rüya–Daniela Kocalevent in a German study[12]. They rated the responses 1-7 from "No, I disagree" to "I agree completely."). The total score is between seven and seventy-seven. In the German study, the average total score was 59.65

The total scores are as follows:

Dr. Emily Spitz: 68
Dr. James Bhat: 57
Miguel Hernandez: 74
Sandra Orozco: 77
Barbara Richardson: 61

The full results are as follows:

Dr. Emily Spitz (total score 68)

1) When I make plans, I follow through with them: **I agree (6)**
2) I usually manage one way or another: **I agree strongly (7)**
3) Keeping interested in things is important to me: **I agree (6)**
4) I feel that I can handle many things at one time: **I agree (6)**
5) I am friends with myself: **I agree (6)**
6) I am determined: I agree strongly (7)
7) I keep an interest in things: **I agree (7)**
8) I can usually find something to laugh about: **I agree (6)**
9) I can look at a situation in a number of ways: **I agree (6)**
10) Sometimes, I make myself do things whether I want to or not: **I agree (6)**

11) I have enough energy to do what I want to do: **I agree** (6)

Dr. James Bhat (total score 57)

1) When I make plans, I follow through with them: **I agree somewhat (5)**
2) I usually manage one way or another: **I agree (6)**
3) Keeping interested in things is important to me: **I agree somewhat (5)**
4) I feel that I can handle many things at one time: **I agree somewhat (5)**
5) I am friends with myself: **undecided/neutral (4)**
6) I am determined: **I agree (6)**
7) I keep an interest in things: **I agree somewhat (5)**
8) I can usually find something to laugh about: **I agree somewhat (5)**
9) I can look at a situation in a number of ways: **I agree (6)**
10) Sometimes, I make myself do things whether I want to or not: **undecided/neutral (4)**
11) I have enough energy to do what I want to do: **I agree (6)**

Miguel Hernandez (total score 74)

1) When I make plans, I follow through with them: **I agree strongly (7)**
2) I usually manage one way or another: **I agree strongly (7)**
3) Keeping interested in things is important to me: **I agree strongly (7)**
4) I feel that I can handle many things at one time: **I agree (6)**
5) I am friends with myself: **I agree strongly (7)**
6) I am determined: I agree strongly (7)
7) I keep an interest in things: **I agree (6)**

8) I can usually find something to laugh about: **I agree strongly (7)**

9) I can look at a situation in a number of ways: **I agree (6)**

10) Sometimes, I make myself do things whether I want to or not: **I agree strongly (7)**

11) I have enough energy to do what I want to do: **I agree strongly (7)**

Sandra Orozco (total score 77)

1) When I make plans, I follow through with them: **I agree strongly (7)**

2) I usually manage one way or another: **I agree strongly (7)**

3) Keeping interested in things is important to me: **I agree strongly (7)**

4) I feel that I can handle many things at one time: **I agree strongly (7)**

5) I am friends with myself: **I agree strongly (7)**

6) I am determined: I agree strongly (7)

7) I keep an interest in things: **I agree strongly (7)**

8) I can usually find something to laugh about: **I agree strongly (7)**

9) I can look at a situation in a number of ways: **I agree strongly (7)**

10) Sometimes, I make myself do things whether I want to or not: **I agree strongly (7)**

11) I have enough energy to do what I want to do: **I agree strongly (7)**

Barbara Richardson (total score 61)

1) When I make plans, I follow through with them: **I agree (6)**

2) I usually manage one way or another: **I agree somewhat (5)**
3) Keeping interested in things is important to me: **I agree (6)**
4) I feel that I can handle many things at one time: **undecided/neutral (4)**
5) I am friends with myself: **I agree somewhat (5)**
6) I am determined: I agree (6)
7) I keep an interest in things: I agree (6)
8) I can usually find something to laugh about: **I agree strongly (7)**
9) I can look at a situation in a number of ways: **I agree strongly (7)**
10) Sometimes, I make myself do things whether I want to or not: **I agree (6)**
11) I have enough energy to do what I want to do: **I disagree somewhat (3)**

APPENDIX D: PHILOSOPHICAL SIGNIFICANCE OF THE NERVOUS SYSTEM

No one would argue with the nervous system's providence over vision and motor function, but the more subjective aspects of consciousness are just as physiological. We think of these things as being intrinsic, but disease can alter or obliterated them. The mind and the body are one. Descartes was wrong; Spinoza was right. This is in the realm of science, not speculation, and I can give you a concrete example.

One of my patients with MS experienced a sudden change in personality. He was normally mild mannered, quiet, and stoic, but he quickly became restless, active, loquacious, and manic. A constant ear-to-ear grin was plastered across his face. He would stay up long hours and snicker at the slightest jest or irregularity. These strange problems developed over several days. He had many other physical signs of neurological disease, but he did not seem to be concerned about the gravity of his condition. An MRI of his brain revealed a large, active lesion (damaged or abnormal tissue) in the right frontal lobe (Figure 4). The association between mania and lesions in the right frontal lobe is well-known[13]. After being treated with intravenous steroids, he improved dramatically, but he never returned to normal. His affect had permanently changed, though someone who had not known him well previously might not notice.

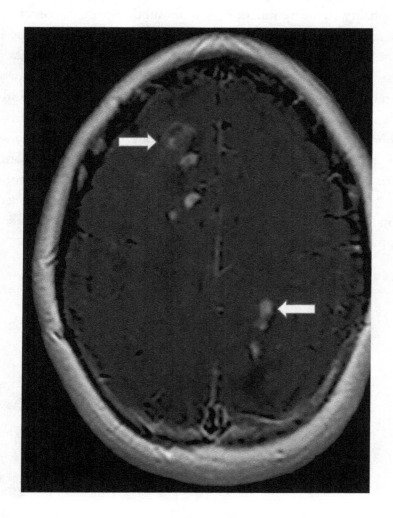

Figure 4. An MRI of the brain, revealing active lesions in the right frontal lobe (toward the left and top of the image), which can cause mania. There are also lesions in the left parietal lobe (to the right and bottom of the image). Note: You are looking from the feet up, so the left side of the brain appears on the right side of the image and vice versa.

I could give you a plethora of other examples of alterations of personality, cognitive function, or other subtle aspects of consciousness related to neurological illnesses. Discrete anatomically localized neurological illnesses can influence sexual orientation,[14] interest in music,[15] and a tendency toward violence. The infamous "Texas tower sniper," Charles Whitman, who murdered seventeen people in a mass shooting in 1966, was found to have a pecan-sized malignant tumor in the right temporal–occipital lobe.[16] Experts concluded that the "tumor conceivably could have contributed to his inability to control his emotions and actions."[16] Dr. Oliver Sacks' book, *The Man Who Mistook His Wife for a Hat and Other Clinical Tales*[17] contains further beautifully written descriptions of interesting neurological conditions.

APPENDICES REFERENCES

1. SoCalSun. BS/MD Results for Class of 2012. College Confidential, 2012 April. Available at http://talk.college-confidential.com/multiple-degree-programs/1300355-bs-md-results-for-class-of-2012-p2.html.

2. 214 Cal.App.4th 921; Court of Appeal, Second District, Division 3, California. The PEOPLE EX REL. Kamala D. HARRIS, as Attorney General, etc., Plaintiff and Appellant, v. Robert A. RIZZO et al., Defendants and Respondents.; B236246; Filed March 20, 2013.

3. 209 Cal.App.4th 93; Court of Appeal, Second District, Division 3, California.; Pier'Angela SPACCIA, Petitioner, v. The SUPERIOR COURT of Los Angeles County, Respondent, People of the State of California, Real Parties in Interest. No. B239472.; Sept. 6, 2012.; As Modified Sept. 25, 2012.

4. Gov.Code, § 36516, subd. (a)(2)(B).

5. Gottlieb J, Vives R. Is a city manager worth $800,000? *LA Times*, July, 15 2010.

6. Medina R, Tuaua AD, Kirk-Gallardo M. County of Los Angeles Maywood City special reelection Maywood City Recall. Los Angeles County Registrar-Recorder/County Clerk, December 9,2008. Available at https://www.lavote.net/documents/dec-9-2008-statement-of-votes-cast.pdf.

7. Gottlieb J, Yoshino K, Vives R. Bell doubled public service taxes and funneled $1 million to Rizzo, audit finds; The doubling of sewer, trash and other service taxes occurred without voter approval. State auditors have spent weeks reviewing the city's financial records. *LA Times*, September 23, 2010.

8. Knoll C, Mather K. Former Bell official Angela Spaccia gets 11 years, 8 months in prison. *LA Times*, April 10, 2014.

9. Jahad S. Sentenced to 12 years in state prison, $9 million in restitution. *KPCC with Associated Press*, April 16 2014.

10. Los Angeles Times Staff. Bell Corruption verdicts. LA Times, March 20, 2013.

11. Knoll C. Former Bell Councilwoman Teresa Jacobo gets two-year prison sentence. *LA Times*, July 25, 2014.

12. Rothe AVE, Zenger M, Lacruz ME, Emeny R, Baumert J, Haefner S, Ladwig KH. Validation and development of a shorter version of the resilience scale RS-11: results from the population-based KORA–age study. *MC Psychology* 2013, 1:25.

13. Joseph R. Frontal lobe psychopathology: mania, depression, confabulation, catatonia, perseveration, obsessive compulsions, and schizophrenia. Psychiatry 1999;62(2):138–172.

14. Wallis L. The stroke had turned me gay. BBC News April 17, 2012.

15. Piore A. When brain damage unlocks the genius within. Pop Sci February 19, 2013.

16. Texas Governor's Committee and Consultants. Report to the Governor, Medical Aspects, Charles J. Whitman Catastrophe. *September 8, 1966.* Available at http://alt.cimedia.com/statesman/specialreports/whitman/findings.pdf. Accessed March, 2016.

17. Sacks O. The Man Who Mistook His Wife for a Hat and Other Clinical Tales. New York: Summit Books, 1985.

ACKNOWLEDGEMENTS

I WOULD LIKE TO thank all of the incredible people living with MS who inspired me to write this book, especially the five people I interviewed: Dr. Emily Spitz, Dr. James Bhat, Sandra Orozco, Miguel Hernandez, and Barbara Richardson. To those living with MS and their caregivers. The MS community on twitter for providing inspiration and encouragement. Medical professionals and researchers sacrificing every day to deliver care to those with MS and to advance the field to improve lives for generations to come. My wife, Elana Beaber, who put up with my writing obsession for five years. My sister, Dr. Sky-Ellen Beaber, who wrote the foreword and gave me invaluable advice and resources. My father, Dr. Rex Julian Beaber, who helped me with Chapters One and Five and introduced me to the brilliant work of Dr. Albert Ellis and Dr. Viktor Frankl. Dr. Mark Katz, author of *Children Who Fail at School but Succeed at Life* who met me in person and helped me with Chapters One and Eleven after I cold-called him. Dr. Melissa Fledderjohann and Dr. John Forsyth who helped me with the Acceptance and Commitment Therapy (ACT) section of Chapter Five. Dr. Annette Langer-Gould who introduced me to the field of MS and is my mentor and colleague. My mentors at The University of Southern California during my fellowship training: Dr. Margaret Burnett,

Dr. Leslie Weiner, Dr. Regina Berkovich, and Dr. Liliana Amezcua. The neurologists at Los Angeles Medical Center essential to my training as a neurology resident including Dr. Sonja Potrebic, Dr. Jane Hwang, Dr. Rani Gowrinathan, Dr. Richard Green, Dr. Larry Rusheen, Dr. Dean Sarco, Dr. Zahra Ajani, Dr. Navdeep Sangha, Dr. Nazanin Matloubi, Dr. Prasanth Manthena, Dr. Bruce Enos, Dr. Jingitan Wang, and Dr. Joseph Chung. To my friend who provided insights about his experience with ALS, Dr. Robert Arbuckle. Dr. Barbara Giesser who gave feedback on the book. Alice Handel, my mother who proofread the manuscript twice. Dr. Alan Epstein who edited the manuscript. J.R. Alcoyne J.D., an amazing beta-reader and author of *Five Fathoms Beneath*. My beta reader Calli who is the director of eQuality, an organization in Minnesota which helps people with disabilities find jobs. Shalom Rabizadeh who helped edit Chapter Six. Editing from The Artful Editor. Early editing from the following accounts on fiverr.com: gingermaneditor, thornecomm5r, kitd56. Donna Rich for final proofreading. 100covers. com for formatting and cover design. Joe Rusko, acquisitions editor at John's Hopkins University Press Health and Wellness division. Dr. Aaron Boster for his incredible passion and activism on social media. Dr. Gavin Giovannoni for his enlightening MS-blogging. The National MS Society (especially Katelyn Michtich and Christian Starks) for giving me the opportunity to interact with the MS community in Southern California. Marie Heron, host of the Living with MS Truth be Told podcast, who interviewed me multiple times. Jon Strum who provides encouragement and information with the RealTalkMS podcast, Yvette Brisco, an MS health coach who interviewed me about neuroplasticity. Dr. Gail C Brady who reviewed the book. My colleagues at Kaiser Downey who have treated me like family, Dr. Henry Lin, Dr. William Miller, Dr. Shelly Bose, Dr. Celine Robinson, Dr. Daniel Ree, Dr. Lidia Tiplea, Dr. James Wei, Maria Higwit, Dr. David Tabby who was my neurology clerkship director in medical school. The many others involved in my education and training.

INDEX

T

U